GUIDE TO POSTGRADUATE
MEDICAL EDUCATION

GUIDE TO POSTGRADUATE MEDICAL EDUCATION

Brian D Keighley,
General Practitioner, Balfron, Stirlingshire

Stuart Murray,
Professor of General Practice, University of Glasgow

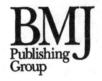

© BMJ Publishing Group 1996

First printed in 1996
by the BMJ Publishing Group, BMA House, Tavistock Square,
London WC1H 9JR

British Library Cataloguing in Publication Data

A catalogue record for this book is available
from the British Library

ISBN 0 7279 – 1072 – 8

Contents

Preface

In the last decade it has been obvious to all doctors that the pace of change within medical practice has accelerated steadily year on year. This is particularly so since the end of the second world war, and medical graduates can no longer expect that their basic medical training will suffice for more than a few short years beyond the completion of training.

It is for this reason that postgraduate education and training is now absolutely intrinsic to the proper professional development of doctors and to the safety of patient care. The traditional medium of education has been the medical textbook, but change is now progressing at a rate that ensures that such textbooks are virtually out of date by the time written material is ready for publication. One theme of this book is to recognise newer methods of disseminating information that rely more on information technology, interactive learning and "learning by doing".

Though technical innovation produces change most quickly within the medical "specialties", general practitioners must have a working knowledge of changing practices so that they can refer appropriately and be capable of undertaking the continuing care of patients on their return to the community.

Vocational training for general practice and continuing medical education for established general practitioners, therefore, have faced enormous challenges in the past few years to fulfil new demands on the educational process. These demands have produced a structure which is almost byzantine in its complexity, is beset by a collection of obscure acronyms, and is an educational maze through which most general practitioners find it almost impossible to navigate.

This book is an attempt to provide a map for that maze. The

most important national organisations concerned are described, together with an analysis of their funding and their affiliations to the two representative bodies of general practice – the Royal College of General Practitioners and the General Medical Services Committee of the BMA. In a more local context the important contributions of regional educational structures, local medical committees, and the medical faculties of universities are described.

Change in medical practice has been accompanied more recently by fundamental change in the NHS and in the general practitioner contract. An attempt has been made to circumscribe these changes, as well as those generated by the General Medical Council, the European Community, and the recent Calman report, all of which promise fresh challenges to general practitioners. Finally, we have made a speculative foray into the future that lies beyond the millennium.

We have already alluded to the fact that the proper organisation of postgraduate medical education is dependent on an amalgam of "academic" and "service" interests, and the credentials of the authors of this book reflect the spirit of the growing cooperation of those two wings of general practice activity.

Whatever develops in the next few years it is clear that the status quo will not remain. The key to "managing" that change will be doctors from the Royal College of General Practitioners and the universities working in harmony with those from the General Medical Services Committee/Local Medical Committee axis. We sincerely hope that this book will be seen as helping that process.

Though morale within general practice is low at the time of writing, there is no doubt that the privilege of being the personal physician to a defined population is still an exciting prospect for a young doctor. This is especially so now with the recognition that general practice is a specialty in its own right, with its own corpus of knowledge and skill. The future health of our discipline can only be enhanced by general practitioners' increasing enthusiasm for education that extends from graduation until retirement, and the restoration of morale will be as dependent on that factor alone as any other.

Every succeeding generation worries about those who come behind – our examination of family doctors' interest and involvement in postgraduate activity leaves us more confident about the future than many other contemporary commentators.

Brian D Keighley
T Stuart Murray
January 1996

Foreword

Postgraduate education is developing and changing rapidly. General practitioners have led the field, and they are to be congratulated on the way in which they have ensured that such initiatives are educationally sound.

The authors describe this book as an attempt to provide a "map for the maze". This is a particularly appropriate analogy as concept mapping is in itself an important educational device. Applied to the general practitioner it suggests the need for detailed knowledge of a number of common conditions and how to manage them most appropriately. This is analogous to the towns, villages, and streets on a map. It also demands, however, that the general practitioner knows a considerable amount about rarer problems. In other words, what goes on in other areas (countries) and in particular how to get there if she needs to. Finally the general practitioner's work is linked to a number of other broader but related disciplines such as education and social services. This takes the map analogy into more distant, but related continents.

In addition to a map, the general practitioner needs a gazetteer. A number of acronyms appear in the book such as AGMETS, COPMED, CRAGPIE, MCQ, OSCE, COG, SCOPME, JCPTGP and these are described allowing the reader to explore and to discover, providing a compass for the way forward.

The educational base of changing general practice has already been mentioned. Education and training are important though the words have slightly different meanings. In the future GPs will need not only to be trained to deal with particular diseases or illnesses, but to be educated to think beyond their own expertise and continually keep up to date. The importance of continuing education and continuing professional development perhaps pose the greatest challenges to the profession as a whole.

Educational methodologies and technical innovations in postgraduate medical education are also of great importance, together with the role of new information systems and their appropriateness in improving the way doctors learn. At the heart of this is the importance of teaching the teachers and ensuring that the quality of the learning experience is tailored to meet individual needs and knowledge. Central to all of this, and emphasised throughout the book, are the values that are held by those in general practice. These values, as exemplified within the General Medical Council's recent documents, set the importance of standards and competence, and emphasise the values of the future general practitioner.

It is important that we do not forget the purpose of this whole process. It is not simply occupational therapy for doctors, or the acquisition of a series of degrees, diplomas or fellowships. It is to provide optimum care for patients and the community involving patients in the process of educating tomorrow's general practitioners.

K C CALMAN
Chief Medical Officer

1 The origins of postgraduate medical education

In the first half of this century medical education in Britain was organised almost totally on "the apprenticeship model", where the student learned informally from a variety of teachers who possessed no special teaching skills. This was most apparent in undergraduate education, but the same principles applied in postgraduate training and education.

Five important documents have changed or promise to change general practitioner education (box 1.1).

Box 1.1 Instruments of change

- Goodenough report (1944)
- Todd report (1968)
- Future general practitioner (1972)
- Tomorrow's doctors (GMC) (1993)
- Calman report (1993–5)

The major impetus for change came from the Royal Commission on Medical Education (the Todd report), which was announced in June 1965, and reported in April 1968. The main recommendations of the report for postgraduate medical education are summarised in box 1.2.

> **Box 1.2 Main recommendations of the Todd report for postgraduate medical education**
>
> - The concept of all doctors, including general practitioners, being specialists in their own field
> - An agreed pattern of professional training for all specialties
> - A new hospital career structure, and the introduction of vocational registration
> - The acceptance that the primary medical degree is no longer recognised as the end point of training, only of basic medical education
> - The establishment of an organisational structure for the delivery of postgraduate medical education

Doctors as specialists

In the mid-1960s a crisis in morale among general practitioners culminated in the 1966 general practitioner charter. Until that time general practice had declined in importance and influence due to two main factors – under-resourcing of staff and premises and general practitioners' professional isolation from the mainstream of hospital medicine. Symptomatic of that low morale was the fact that postgraduate medical education was largely bypassing family medicine, despite the fact that 90% of all illnesses have always been treated in that environment.

The Todd report looked into the future and examined models in other countries where family medicine had all but disappeared in favour of specialisation, notably in North America. It based its recommendations, however, on the premise that there would still be a need for a family doctor service centred on communities, and it correctly predicted the pattern of medical care that has emerged in the United Kingdom of the 1990s. Todd also correctly predicted the demise of the single handed practitioner in favour of group practice and the formation of the primary health care team.

Todd's view of general practitioner specialisation was that of a large group of general practitioners working in association, each practitioner becoming a "specialist in the community" and developing a special skill in only one specialty. A working model did develop in the practice attached to the new town of Livingston on the outskirts of Edinburgh in the early 1970s. Though general practitioners are slowly usurping the role of hospitals' general

---

Box 1.3 The knowledge, skills and attitudes of general practice (1972)

At the conclusion of the training programme, the doctor should be able to demonstrate:

I Knowledge

that he has sufficient knowledge of disease processes, particularly of common diseases, chronic diseases and those which endanger life or have serious complications or consequences;

that he understands the opportunities, methods and limitations of prevention, early diagnosis and management in the setting of general practice;

his understanding of the way in which interpersonal relationships within the family can cause health problems or alter their presentation, course and management, just as illness can influence family relationships;

an understanding of the social and environmental circumstances of his patients, and how they may affect a relationship between health and illness;

his knowledge and appropriate use of the wide range of interventions available to him;

that he understands the ethics of his profession and their importance for the patient;

that he understands the basic methods of research as applied to general practice;

an understanding of medico-social legislation and the impact of this on his patient.

II Skills

how to form diagnoses which take account of physical, psychological and social factors;

that he understands the use of epidemiology and probability in his everyday work;

understanding and use of the factor 'time' as a diagnostic, therapeutic and organisational tool;

that he can identify persons at risk and take appropriate action;

that he can make relevant initial decisions about every problem presented to him as a doctor;

the capacity to cooperate with medical and non-medical professionals;

knowledge and appropriate use of the skills of practice management.

III Attitudes

a capacity for empathy and for forming a specific and effective relationship with patients and for developing a degree of self understanding;

how his recognition of the patient as a unique individual modifies the ways in which he elicits information and makes hypotheses about the nature of his problems and their management;

that he understands that helping patients to solve their own problems is a fundamental therapeutic activity;

that he recognises that he can make a professional contribution to the wider community;

that he is willing and able critically to evaluate his own work;

that he recognises his own need for continuing education and critical reading of medical information.

---

physicians, however, specialism in general practice has not followed Todd's concept. General practitioners have not become paediatricians or dermatologists, rather they have become experts in primary care medicine, which is now recognised as a specialty in its own right.

The attributes required for the specialist in primary care were documented in the Royal College of General Practitioners' 1972 publication *The Future General Practitioner*, which described five areas of knowledge required of the modern general practitioner and it is still cited today as the template for the educational curriculum of the rounded general practitioner.

The five areas it described were clinical practice – health and diseases; clinical practice – human development; clinical practice – human behaviour; medicine and society; and the practice.

Thus, for the first time it was clearly stated that the job of a British general practitioner included the physical, mental, and social aspects of health and disease and not merely the treatment of episodes of illness.

Two important conferences took place in Leeuwenhorst in the Netherlands in 1972 and 1974, each of which produced an important declaration, *The Knowledge, Skills and Attitudes of General Practice* (1972) and *The Role of the General Practitioner* (1974). These seminal statements are reproduced in boxes 1.3 and 1.4.

Box 1.4 The role of the general practitioner (1974)

The general practitioner is a licensed medical graduate who gives personal, primary and continuing care to individuals, families and a practice population, irrespective of age, sex and illness; it is the synthesis of these functions which is unique. He will attend his patients in his consulting room and in their homes and sometimes in a clinic or hospital. His aim is to make early diagnoses. He will include and integrate physical, psychological and social factors in his considerations about health and illness. This will be expressed in the care of his patients. He will make an initial decision about every problem which is presented to him as a doctor. He will undertake the continuing management of his patients with chronic, recurrent or terminal illnesses. Prolonged contact means that he can use repeated opportunities to gather information at a pace appropriate to each patient, and build up a relationship of trust which he can use professionally. He will practice in cooperation with other colleagues, medical and non-medical. He will know when to intervene through treatment, prevention and education, to promote the health of his patients and their families. He will recognise that he also has a professional responsibility to the community.

The concept of the general practitioner as a specialist in primary care has made many demands of postgraduate training and education and has been the main engine of change in the postgraduate field over the past 30 years.

Agreed pattern of training for all specialties

Currently there is great change under way within British medicine and the NHS, and those concerned with medical education agree that four different phases of that education should be defined. The Todd report's findings were remarkably prescient, and the four phases of today's education were defined as far back as 1968; they are:

- The intern year which corresponds to the preregistration year, when fledgling doctors adapt to the change in role from medical student, taking more responsibility for patient management under supervised conditions, but at the same time still acquiring basic clinical skills
- General professional training lasting about three years, when doctors acquire the knowledge and skills in the general area of their intended career
- Further professional training which is a transitional phase between that of training for a specialty and that of gradually taking on board those responsibilities that will equip them for independent practice in their chosen career
- Continuing medical education and training – a process for all career grade doctors to allow them to refresh their knowledge and keep abreast of new developments.

New hospital career structure and the introduction of vocational registration

In 1993 the chief medical officer published proposals for a new career structure for hospital training grades in response to the requirements of the European Directives, the eponymous Calman report, which is fully described in chapter 12. In this area, also, the Todd report predicted the need for change by recommending a grading structure that largely corresponds to that of Sir Kenneth Calman in the 1990s – junior house officer leading to full registration, senior house officer during basic professional training, and a unified training grade for further professional training. Todd also predicted the grade of "specialist" from which entry to the ranks of consultant would be sought. Allied with this plan was the additional concept of vocational registration which corresponds to Calman's certificate of completion of specialist training (CCST).

The status of the primary medical degree

In 1944 the Goodenough committee recommended that a medical graduate should not be allowed full registration until he or she had held two six month approved house officer posts in medicine and surgery. Legislation to give effect to these proposals was enacted in 1950, but until 1953 it was still possible for the young doctor to be "capped" on the Saturday and for the newly fledged graduate to start work as a principal general practitioner on the next Monday morning.

As the complexity and scope of medical training has increased over the past 50 years it has become obvious that the primary medical degree is but a stepping stone from a very basic grounding in medical practice to the more intensive and focused training that a doctor receives in his or her first years in practice.

Tomorrow's Doctors, published by the General Medical Council (GMC) in 1993 goes even further in demoting the primary medical degree as any form of "end point" to training. It has pointed out the increasing "factual overload" that has been visited on medical students in recent years and recommends that this should be reduced drastically. Rather than impart a raft of facts to students the new model of undergraduate education will be still to teach a "core curriculum" of essential knowledge, skills and attitudes. This core curriculum will be supplemented by a series of "special study modules" which will allow students to develop new areas of study of their own choice that will guide them in *how* to learn rather than giving a prescriptive list of facts that must be learnt by all.

As its second principal recommendation, *Tomorrow's Doctors* states " . . . the undergraduate course should be seen as the first stage in the continuum of medical education that extends throughout professional life".

The organisational structure for the delivery of postgraduate medical education

At the time of writing the organisation of postgraduate medical education is facing yet another major upheaval as adaptations are made to that proposed by Todd in the 1960s. These changes are to align educational structures with the new organisation of the NHS and the purchaser-provider split brought in by the government in 1989-90. Whatever structure eventually emerges, however, it will be built on the foundations laid by Todd 30 years ago.

Before 1965 the organisation of postgraduate education was splintered between a number of bodies, a situation that had developed for historical reasons rather than one that had been planned for. Todd recognised that postgraduate education was of great mutual importance to three groups of organisations; the professional bodies (notably the medical royal colleges), the NHS, and the universities.

Todd recommended that a central body was needed with tripartite representation which would:

- Ensure a comprehensive scheme for postgraduate professional training for all specialties, including general practice
- Ensure sufficient training posts were available
- Ensure a training scheme in each and every region
- Ensure assessment of general professional training
- Ensure continuing medical education was organised both nationally and regionally
- Ensure proper arrangements for overseas doctors coming to the United Kingdom for training
- Ensure an exchange of ideas between the regions that kept all concerned abreast of educational developments.

It is precisely these same aims and objectives that are driving the current changes in the structure of postgraduate education.

The central bodies established in the 1960s were the national councils of postgraduate medical education. The English council was disbanded in 1988, but the councils for Wales and Northern Ireland survive. Uniquely, the Scottish council was reconstituted

7

as a special health authority in 1994 and had dentistry added to its remit. Perhaps the most important innovation, however, was the establishment of a structure below that of the national councils, and regional committees of postgraduate medical education were set up together with the new offices of postgraduate medical dean and regional adviser in general practice.

The regional committees, together with their executive officers, have been the building blocks of an effective postgraduate organisation over the past three decades, and while adaptations will be described later, this structure has served British medicine and its patients well and is likely to continue into the next century in a similar form even after the current government has brought in measures to increase managerial and financial accountability along the currently fashionable perceptions of how to organise activity in the public sector.

Summary

Postgraduate medical education in Britain has developed under the influence of several institutions, but notably the medical royal colleges and other professional bodies, the NHS, and the universities. These disparate elements have been woven into a national structure for the United Kingdom because of the publication of a few important documents whose influence has stood the test of time and of change in the health delivery system. Further change is still planned. The fundamental principles on which postgraduate education is founded, with the recognition that patient care is paramount and that the study of medicine is a lifelong pursuit, have ensured that new and changing structures should continue to meet its needs into the next century.

General practice has been the discipline that has undergone the most change over the past 50 years. General practice is supposed to be "pivotal" to the reformed NHS, and therefore its involvement in postgraduate education and in shaping educational policy and its implementation has never been more important.

Further reading

Royal Commission on Medical Education. *Report (Todd report)*. London: HMSO, 1968.

Interdepartmental Committee on Medical Schools. *Report (Goodenough report)*. London: HMSO, 1944.

Royal College of General Practitioners. *The future general practitioner: learning and teaching*. London: British Medical Journal, 1972. (Republished 1990, RCGP.)

General Medical Council. *Tomorrow's Doctors*. London: GMC, 1993.

Calman K. *Hospital doctors: training for the future. The report of the working group on specialist medical training*. London: Health Publications Unit, 1993.

Calman K. *Hospital doctors: training for the future. The report of the working group on specialist medical training. A supplementary report by the working group commissioned to consider the implications for general medical practice arising from the principal report*. London: Health Publications Unit, 1994.

Royal College of General Practitioners. The story of postgraduate education. In: *Forty years on: the story of the first forty years of the RCGP*. London: RCGP, 1992.

2 The structure of general practitioner postgraduate education

As with most frameworks applied to the medical profession that for postgraduate medical education is hierarchical. Most descriptions of a hierarchy are given in a "top down" fashion, but this book is written for general practitioners and therefore there is a certain logic in beginning at the level of the individual general practitioner and relating the whole edifice of a complicated structure to the basic unit of a practice where there are one or more

---

Box 2.1 Postgraduate medical education: individuals and organisations relating to the General Practitioner Practice, Principal, and General Practitioner Registrar.

- General practitioner trainer
- Primary health care team
- Local vocational training scheme and its course organiser (associate adviser in Scotland)
- Local hospital consultants
- Postgraduate tutor
- Family health services authority general manager (primary care manager of the health board in Scotland)
- Local medical committee (area general practitioner subcommittee in Sotland)
- Local faculty of the royal college
- Local clinical audit committee

---

general practitioner principals and, possibly, a vocational trainee (general practitioner registrar).

Those individuals and organisations which relate to postgraduate medical education and the general practitioner practice are summarised in box 2.1.

The general practitioner trainer

In a training practice it is the trainer who has traditionally carried responsibility for education, but it is now thought that the entire practice should be a training environment for the general practitioner vocational trainee (GP registrar) and all partners should be concerned. It is still true, however, that the designated trainer often takes the lead and is the partner to whom both registrars and partners will turn on educational matters. Indeed, in Scotland, the post of trainer is seen as an academic appointment by invitation. An appointed trainer receives a training grant in recognition of his or her work which forms part of the average intended net remuneration for general practitioners, but the trainee's salary and allowances are centrally funded.

Though quality is by no means *confined* to training practices, there is no doubt that their rigorous selection and reaccreditation should ensure that training practices are of the highest standard. For this reason trainers are often active in the postgraduate education of other principals and are called on to offer their skill in a wider forum locally than that concerned with their own practice or training scheme.

Certain attributes are demanded of trainers, and local training schemes are responsible and answerable for trainer selection within nationally set parameters. Just as with practices, these qualities are not *exclusive* to trainers, but such appointments should still be seen as a mark of distinction in a discipline that has always eschewed any form of pecking order in its structure.

The primary health care team

With the development of the team concept of care within general practice, members of *other* disciplines are often now able to offer education and training opportunities.

Nurses, midwives, and health visitors work in ever closer cooperation with doctors in the community, and their unique perspectives on community health problems have become useful additions to the educational resource available to general practice.

11

This is not to say that general practitioners are now to abandon a leadership role nor to change their educational priorities; but in a discipline that advances a holistic approach, such insights from associated professions should not be ignored.

Similarly, opportunities arise from the professions allied to medicine and, if prejudice can be overcome, there are often useful educational inputs from other caring cultures, such as social work.

Management within general practice has never been more important, especially with the introduction of the 1990 contract, and a skilled and knowledgeable practice manager is also a resource for inexperienced general practitioners and for registrars.

The vocational training scheme and the course organiser

Once established as the points of reference for education within practices or localities, GP trainers have a need for their own personal development and mutual support. The local vocational training scheme provides a framework for such support. GP trainers are either attached to local schemes where registrars fulfil certain preordained hospital jobs, with a GP trainer already chosen, or they offer their posts to registrars who are constructing their own programmes of training. In both cases, however, trainers organise themselves into local groups and meet together, usually monthly, to discuss educational methods, problems, and innovations.

The "leader" of this group of trainers, the course organiser, is chosen for proved academic talent but also for skill in acting as a facilitator and mentor to others. It is to this figure that trainers will turn first with educational problems, be they personal, professional, or related to a difficulty with a registrar. The success of training and education in any local area is often dependent on the quality of the course organiser and his or her ability effectively to organise education among an intelligent and strong minded peer group. (The course organiser is known as the associate adviser in general practice in Scotland.)

Local hospital consultants

With notable exceptions, the input of hospital consultants to general practitioner education had a notorious reputation in the past for boring, didactic, and irrelevant lectures delivered to a reluctant audience which was there solely to gain credit for payment of seniority allowances!

Consultants have always had an important contribution to make to the education of registrars, however; indeed two of the three years of prescribed vocational training are under the tutelage of just such hospital doctors.

The development of community based consultants in disciplines such as paediatrics, mental health, and geriatrics has produced a newer breed of doctors who have a considerable contribution to make to general practitioners' education. In addition, where outreach clinics have been established by consultants in general practitioners' own premises (often as a result of fundholding) educational opportunities have arisen for principals which are the more valuable because they are related to real patients with real problems.

The postgraduate tutor

Most hospital doctors have teaching responsibilities as an integral part of their professional lives, even though many are not specifically selected for the role nor have they been trained in educational methods. This contrasts starkly with general practitioner trainers. The doctors with prime responsibility for developing and fostering this education within hospitals are the postgraduate tutors.

The postgraduate tutors are academic appointments made by universities through the deans and regional committees and have administrative responsibility for unit educational budgets delegated from postgraduate deans. All hospital training grades come under the supervision of postgraduate tutors, who also organise the administration and financing of local postgraduate centres.

They must organise their work in the knowledge that half of the young doctors for whom they are responsible will eventually end up in general practice. It is essential, therefore, that a close working relationship and professional understanding is developed between postgraduate tutors and course organisers.

Postgraduate tutors also have responsibilities for continuing medical education (CME) and many general practitioner principals will come to know their local postgraduate tutors as respected, local educators.

The family health services authority general manager

The family health services authority (FHSA) has the responsibility to arrange for the salary and allowances for registrars. It also has to ensure that the general practitioner has fulfilled the continuing medical education requirements for payment of the postgraduate educational allowance. Such managers, therefore, have a peripheral but important administrative and financial role in general practitioner education, and no description of such education would be complete without mention of them and paragraphs 37 and 38 of the statement of fees and allowances (SFA).

The local medical committee (LMC)

The local medical committee impinges on general practitioner education because of its duty to nominate a member who is representative of all local general practitioners to the regional committees which choose trainers and which regulate regional educational policy relating to training schemes. These committees have an additional educational role for general practitioners and registrars alike in relation to prescribing matters, service committees, and the interpretation of the byzantine intricacies of the statement of fees and allowances.

The local faculty of the Royal College of General Practitioners (RCGP)

The RCGP also nominates members to regional postgraduate committees and is therefore of equal importance in the formulation of local and regional educational policy. It is also the general practitioner body most concerned with education and standards and, of course, sets the only professional examination relating to the discipline – the MRCGP. The role of the college and its examination is explored more fully in a later chapter.

The local clinical audit committee

Clinical audit is *not* strictly postgraduate medical education, but it is certainly a closely allied pursuit. Currently evidence based medicine is becoming important in both practice and in education, and clinical audit is one of the main building blocks for the compilation of such evidence. An awareness of the principles of clinical audit is a requirement for all GP registrars and is increasingly so for the fully developed general practitioner.

The membership of clinical audit committees is multidisciplinary and is in the gift of local health authorities. The general practitioner membership of this committee, however, will normally include input from the local medical committee, the royal college, and GP purchasers. Any general practitioner interested in postgraduate education would be well advised to be aware of the influence on it of clinical audit.

Regional structures

Once the general practitioner principal acquires an understanding of local educational organisation it is important that he or she also understands how it relates to that at regional level, because decisions made at the region have a significant bearing on how matters are arranged locally.

Those individuals and organisations that operate at regional level are summarised in box 2.2.

Box 2.2 Postgraduate medical education: individuals and organisations at regional level

- Regional adviser in general practice
- Regional postgraduate education committee and its general practitioner subcommittees
- Regional postgraduate dean (or director)

The regional adviser in general practice

The regional advisers are key players in the organisation of general practitioners' postgraduate medical education. Not only are they central to the operation of vocational training schemes but they have a role in the continuing medical education of their principal peers. Originally it was thought essential that regional advisers should fulfil their educational role on a part time basis so that they should remain exposed to the realities of the day to day general medical practice, better to understand the aims of the education they oversee. As the job has increased in scope and complexity, however, their clinical exposure has become much less and some advisers in the larger regions have only minimal exposure to patients. Indeed, as will be seen later, many are soon to change their status to that of civil servant. At the moment they are appointed by universities, recognised by the royal college, and have their salaries reimbursed by health authorities.

Regional advisers have several advisory roles. Primarily they advise the region's chief executive officer for postgraduate education, the postgraduate dean (or director); they advise the regional Postgraduate Medical Education Committee; and they are available to give advice and guidance to all those who are in training or who aspire to a general practice career.

The Calman report has recommended new financial responsibilities for regional advisers, and it seems likely that they are soon to become the budget holders and the "purchasers" of general practitioner education.

The qualities demanded of these doctors are many and complicated. It is essential that they command the respect of general practitioner principals as competent and caring clinicians; as many have university credentials and are active within the royal college – they must have intellectual and academic credibility; and with new purchasing responsibilities they must have managerial and financial skills. In addition, it is important that they are seen as even handed in their treatment of all connected with general practice, showing professional integrity and a balanced approach to the competing priorities of education, doctors' personal development, good patient care, legitimate management objectives, fiscal accountability, and value for money.

As executive officers of the regional structure regional advisers are central to those decisions concerned with trainer selection (and deselection), standards of training, the appointment of course organisers, the standards of hospital training for general practitioners, and continuing medical education for established principals.

Not only do they relate "downwards" to general practitioner principals and registrars and laterally to regional committees and supporting structures, but they are the central point of reference "upwards" to national organisations concerned with training such as the Joint Committee on Postgraduate Training for General Practice (JCPTGP) and other important bodies to be described later in the chapter.

The regional postgraduate dean (or director)

Though the proportion of the NHS budget devoted to

education and training is tiny, the sums of public money handled at regional level in absolute terms are very large, hence the need for professional, managerial, and financial accountability. The regional chief officers who fulfil this function are the postgraduate deans.

They may chair the regional postgraduate education committees, or act as their executive officers, and their salary costs are shared between a university and the health authority (different arrangements apply in Wales, and the Scottish arrangements are described later). They tend to hold full time appointments, and the professional and managerial skills described above for regional advisers are equally important.

They have a wide range of responsibilities for medical education and training, which include both hospital medicine and general practice, the funding of postgraduate medical centres, and for the continuing medical education of all career grade doctors, including the operation of the doctors' retainer scheme. They are the budget holders at regional level for both postgraduate training and continuing medical education.

Regional postgraduate education committees

Since 1991 these committees have been reduced in size and in responsibility. They are primarily there to be advisory to postgraduate deans in discharging their executive functions and are a useful interdisciplinary medical forum where matters of mutual interest are discussed and consensus advice formulated.

It is usual to find subordinate structures associated with these regional committees, and that concerned with general practice will give advice on educational policy, trainer selection, and the fulfilment of minimal educational criteria visited on regions by national regulatory bodies (such as the Joint Committee on Postgraduate Training for General Practice). Regional advisers will also relate to this committee structure for general practice either as chairpersons or executive officers. Both the full regional committee and its subcommittees have representatives from local general practice, usually appointed by local medical committees (area medical committees in Scotland) and by the local faculty of the royal college. Other representatives are drawn from health authorities, public health medicine, postgraduate tutors, and the consultant establishment.

National structures

The organisation of general practitioner education at a national level is sensibly integrated with education of the medical profession as a whole and is within the remit of several powerful all-embracing educational bodies. Other national bodies are exclusively concerned with general practice, and the word "national" can sometimes relate to England and Wales only and sometimes to the whole of the United Kingdom. At the end of this chapter the differences within the United Kingdom are highlighted. The national bodies concerned with general practitioner education are summarised in box 2.3.

The General Medical Council (GMC)

The GMC is the regulatory body for the entire medical profession. It has several committees, some of which are prescribed by the Medical Acts:

• The education committee sets the standard to which universities must comply for undergraduate medical education and inspects their compliance

• The preliminary proceedings committee considers cases of professional misconduct referred to it by one or more

---

Box 2.3 National bodies concerned with general practitioner education and training

• The General Medical Council (GMC)
• Joint Committee on Postgraduate Training for General Practice (JCPTGP)
• Conference of Regional Advisers in General Practice in England (CRAGPIE)
• UK Conference of Regional Advisers in General Practice
• UK Conference of Postgraduate Deans
• Conference of Postgraduate Medical Deans (COPMED)
• Standing Committee on Postgraduate Medical and Dental Education (SCOPME)
• Joint Higher Training Committees (JHTCs)
• Advisory Group on Medical and Dental Education, Training and Staffing (AGMETS)

"preliminary screeners", three medical and two lay; this committee may dispose of a case by a letter of advice or by referral to either the health committee or the professional conduct committee

- The health committee – when a doctor does not cooperate with a "health screener", may direct that a doctor's registration be subject to certain conditions or may direct suspension of registration for a renewable period of 12 months

- The professional conduct committee will decide whether charges of professional misconduct on the part of a doctor are proved and, if so, can conclude the case with an admonition, impose special conditions on a doctor's registration, direct suspension of registration for a renewable period of 12 months, or direct indefinite erasure from the register.

In addition to these "statutory" committees, the GMC appoints members to the following internal bodies:

- The president's advisory committee assists the president in the fulfilment of his or her role relevant to the council's statutory functions and advises particularly on proposed changes to the council's constitution, policy, or functions; essentially, it is an executive inner caucus of the GMC

- The finance and establishment committee considers all matters pertaining to the financial affairs of the GMC

- The overseas committee considers the special questions of the recognition of overseas medical qualifications and the registration of doctors who qualified overseas and who wish to practise in the United Kingdom

- The registration committee is concerned with all matters pertaining to medical registration, which is the sole criterion for practice as a medical practitioner in the United Kingdom

- The committee on standards of professional conduct and on medical ethics compiles a guide and code of practice for all doctors in the United Kingdom, departure from which might well be considered "serious professional misconduct".

The Joint Committee on Postgraduate Training for General Practice is the delegated competent authority for general practice for all doctors originating inside the United Kingdom and the

European Community, but the GMC is the competent authority for the remainder.

With the introduction of new performance procedures the GMC will have important duties with regard to underperforming general practitioners both in assessing their questioned performance and in prescribing any retraining that is required. (The parliamentary bill introducing these new procedures was enacted in the autumn of 1995, and new procedures should be in place by 1997.)

The Joint Committee on Postgraduate Training for General Practice (JCPTGP)

This committee was founded in 1975–6 to monitor the quality of vocational training for general practice which became mandatory for all new entrants under the vocational training regulations of 1979. It issues certificates of prescribed or equivalent experience on satisfactory completion of vocational training. On being appointed the "competent authority" under European legislation in 1995 it was given the additional responsibility of supervising the actual training given and, as such, is the professional educational authority for United Kingdom graduates for entry to general practice.

The membership of the committee is drawn principally from the royal college and the GMSC, but there is also representation from the Joint Consultants Committee and various medical education interests, and it includes observers from standing medical education committees and from the health departments.

Its main function is to certify experience as having been satisfactorily completed, and no doctor can become a principal on a medical list without such a certificate. In addition it has the duty to provide advice to aspiring general practitioners as to how to achieve its certificate.

Its main standard setting function is carried out by periodic inspection of training standards operated by regions throughout the United Kingdom in both hospital training posts and the general practice year, and from time to time it issues guidance over the minimum standards expected of regions in the vocational training carried out within them. If a region is deemed to be unsatisfactory it is informed of this finding, and such a finding is widely publicised. The final sanction of the committee to refuse recognition has never been tested, neither have the consequences which could flow from such a decision. The threat of public criticism of a region by the committee, however, has so far been sufficient to cause standards to rise to the acceptable.

Conference of Regional Advisers in General Practice in England (CRAGPIE)

The conference of regional advisers was established by the Department of Health in England in 1988 and reviewed in 1991. Its formal remit is "to provide a national forum for regional advisers in general practice to discuss problems of mutual interest among themselves and with colleagues; and to help anybody seeking the advice of the committee on these matters". This forum, therefore, allows discussion and development of policy on postgraduate medical education for general practice, ensuring national consistency for that policy and for high standards of general practitioner training.

The conference is funded from various sources, and its membership includes all English advisers, a Welsh representative, a postgraduate dean, two members from the NHS Executive, and observers from the royal college and the joint committee.

United Kingdom conference of Regional Advisers and United Kingdom conference of Postgraduate Deans

Both these committees were established in 1975. They have no formal terms of reference, but their remit is to relate to all the United Kingdom health departments (England, Wales, Scotland, and Northern Ireland). They deal with changes within the health service and examine educational and research matters but remain separate and distinct from the NHS management.

The membership of the committees is respectively made up of the postgraduate deans and regional advisers from all parts of the United Kingdom. The Department of Health is usually invited to send an observer, and the committees' self funding status is derived from various sources.

Conference of Postgraduate Deans (COPMED)

This committee is analogous in structure, membership, and funding to the conference of regional advisers. It represents only postgraduate deans in England and is funded from their own budget. It meets monthly to pool information, to discuss problems, and to advise the Department of Health and its secretary of state.

Standing Committee on Postgraduate Medical and Dental Education (SCOPME)

This committee is the successor to the Council for Postgraduate Medical Education (for England) which was disbanded in 1988. In 1993 dental education was added to its remit and title. It has the status of a non-departmental public body and was set up under statutory authority (NHS Act 1977).

Its remit is, "to advise the secretary of state on the delivery of postgraduate medical and dental education, taking into account both the standards promulgated by professional and educational bodies and the potential difficulties of reconciling service and training needs; to identify particular problems and to develop realistic solutions to these in consultation with relevant interests and to report regularly".

Thus, this committee is much more of an arm of government than other educational bodies and is constrained to act in accordance with prevailing governmental policy. A line of accountability for all aspects of its work and operation and that of its working groups exists from its chairperson to the secretary of state and ultimately to parliament. The chief executive of the NHS executive acts as the accounting officer, and he or she is also answerable to the parliamentary commissioner for all issues of maladministration.

It is directly funded by the Department of Health and subject to departmental financial audit. Wales comes under its remit but not Scotland (see below).

Joint higher training committees (JHTCs)

These committees are non-statutory bodies that have evolved to ensure that the views of the medical royal colleges and faculties on higher specialist training are turned into practice. The nature, composition, and method of working adopted by each individual body vary; there is a common function, however, to agree standards and programmes of higher specialist training and to approve the posts at specialist registrar level that provide such training.

Funding for the training committees is provided by secretarial support from the colleges and faculties, a grant in aid from the health departments, and travel and subsistence costs for inspection visits from health authorities. Membership is drawn from college representatives, university departments, specialist associations, postgraduate deans, and observers from the health departments. General practice is serviced by the Joint Committee on Postgraduate Training as described above.

Advisory Group on Medical and Dental Education, Training, and Staffing (AGMETS)

This advisory group was set up in 1994 as a single, overarching body to oversee all medical and dental workforce issues within the health service. It oversees *Achieving a Balance*, an initiative to ensure the supply of trained doctors for each specialty, and the implementation of the Calman report, which introduces a new, unified hospital training grade with planned and structured training. The specialist workforce advisory group (SWAG) operates within the structure and advises on the number of higher specialist trainees required for each specialty.

AGMETS membership is drawn from the NHS management, the medical profession in both hospital and general practice, and the Departments of Health for England and Wales. There are observers from SCOPME and the Scottish and Northern Ireland Offices. In 1995 it was agreed that the representation from general practice should be increased and that there should be a dedicated subgroup for the discipline.

Special arrangements for Scotland

The Scottish Council for Postgraduate Medical and Dental Education (SCPMDE) was established in 1994 as a special health authority with the remit to, "stimulate, coordinate, monitor and advise on the development, organisation, funding and delivery of postgraduate and continuing medical and dental education and training in Scotland; distribute the resources provided and ensure the efficiency and effectiveness of their use; and provide a national forum". As an organisation it grew from a previous Scottish council, recommended by the Todd report of 1968, which had survived the review of the English council (which effectively was transformed into SCOPME).

The Scottish council has several distinct features that makes it unique among similar organisations in other parts of the United Kingdom:

- It has the unique status of a health authority and is accountable to government in the same way as all other such authorities

- It has a board of management drawn from the three "stake holders" in postgraduate education; the profession, the universities, and NHS management (both purchasers and providers)

- It holds and distributes 100% of the basic salary costs of all hospital training grades (only 50% is held centrally in England and Wales).

- It ensures that a tripartite "service and training agreement" is in place for all junior hospital doctors, signed by SCPMDE through the postgraduate dean, the employing trust, and the doctors concerned, specifying both the service and training component of each hospital job

- It employs the Scottish postgraduate deans and regional advisers, who are accountable financially and professionally to its executive director

- It distributes and oversees all section 63 funds for the training of GP registrars and their trainers

- It distributes and oversees the funding for postgraduate tutors and postgraduate centres

- It has, in addition, roles in coordination of medical education, implementation and monitoring of educational policy at national and regional levels, clinical audit, educational research and innovation, the education of doctors from overseas and those on the doctors' retainer scheme, provision of career advice, continuing medical education, funding of study leave for hospital doctors in training, and cooperation with other United Kingdom bodies with similar remits

- It has the same terms of reference for postgraduate dental education.

The Scottish council therefore has educational and executive functions, largely mediated through the postgraduate deans, and a regional structure, but manpower issues have been the remit of other bodies, such as the Advisory Committee on Medical Establishments (ACME) for hospitals and the Scottish Medical Practices Committee (SMPC) for general practice.

In 1995 the organisation of medical and dental education in England and Wales was thrown into confusion by the government's decision to abolish the regional tier of NHS management to which educational structures had previously related. The unique position of SCPMDE as a unified and coherent organisation, has avoided this confusion, and it seems strange to those medical educationalists living and working in Scotland that the concept of this single over-arching body has not been exported south of the border, which has representation from all the "stakeholders" in medical education, especially as the wheel seems to have been re-invented there in the shape of Advisory Group on Medical and Dental Education, Training, and Staffing.

In Scotland too, however, an equivalent body to AGMETS has recently been formed. This advisory group is called the Scottish Advisory Committee on the Medical Workforce and supercedes the functions of ACME. As with most features of the NHS, it seems that the Richmond House dog is wagging the St Andrew's House tail!

Further reading

National Association of Health Authorities and Trusts, *Partners in learning: developing postgraduate training and continuing education for general practice*. London: NAHAT, 1994.

Royal College of General Practitioners, *Education and training for general practice*. London: RCGP, 1994.

Secretary of State for Health, *Working for patients: postgraduate and continuing medical and dental education*. London: HMSO, 1989.

UK Health Departments, Joint Consultants Committee, and Chairmen of Regional Health Authorities, *Hospital medical staffing – achieving a balance*. London: Department of Health, 1987.

3 "The ground work" – undergraduate teaching for general practice

The main impetus for undergraduate teaching of general practice came from the college of general practitioners. There is evidence, however, that teaching in general practice was being developed before the college was in existence. A course of six lectures in general practice had taken place in 1935 as an extra for the students at St Mary's Hospital in London. This was a welcome innovation, and the lectures were repeated annually and every second year during the second world war. After the war a full time one week attachment was arranged with a general practitioner and proved popular with the students. Teaching expanded when a teaching practice was set up at the University of Edinburgh in the early 50s, and there were also reports at this time from other parts of the country. The teaching of general practice grew gradually over the next 20 years with the main expansion coming in the early 70s after the publication of the report by the Royal Commission on medical education.

In 1980 the education committee of the GMC strongly recommended a period of attachment to a general practitioner for undergraduate medical students. This attachment would give the student an opportunity to study types of illness not normally requiring hospital treatment in addition to the early and late manifestation of many diseases which are seen in hospital at a different stage. An attachment would also provide first hand knowledge of available community resources for domiciliary care and the promotion of health and allow the observation of general practice as a means of providing continuing care for the patient and family. Finally the student would be able to observe general practice as a vocational opportunity. The GMC recognised that experience in general practice was facilitated where university departments of general practice and teaching practices had been created. The Association of University Teachers in General Practice reported in 1984 that 16 of the 20 GMC recommendations for undergraduate medical education could not be achieved at any reasonable level by students without using the educational resources of general practice. In 1987 a further working party of the GMC education committee stated that some of the priorities in medical education must change to adapt to the changing pattern of disease, a changing population structure, and new technology. Departments of community medicine and general practice with the help of teachers of behavioural sciences could help medicine to respond to these challenges. Teaching of behavioural science since that time has been a partnership involving the departments mentioned.

Box 3.1 Attachment to general practice

- Demonstrates illness not normally seen in hospital
- Early and late manifestations of disease
- First hand knowledge of available community resources
- Means of providing continuing care

Fraser selected 11 objects from the GMC's original list in which he thought that general practice was the appropriate locus for the student to achieve the objectives. (The letters used to denote each objective are those used in the original GMC list.)

- To acquire knowledge and understanding of:

  e) The principles of prevention and of therapy, including health education, the amelioration of suffering and disability, rehabilitation, the maintenance of health in old age, and the care of the dying
  f) Human relationships, both personal and communal, and the interaction between man and his physical, biological, and social environment

- To develop the professional skills necessary:

  a) To elicit, record, and interpret the relevant medical history, symptoms, and physical signs, and to identify the problems and how these may be managed
  c) To deal with common medical emergencies
  d) To communicate effectively and sensitively with patients and their relatives
  f) To use laboratory and other diagnostic and therapeutic services effectively and economically and in the best interests of his patients

- To develop appropriate attitudes to the practice of medicine which include:

  a) Recognition that a blend of scientific and humanitarian approaches is needed in medicine
  b) A capacity for self education so that he may continue to develop and extend knowledge and skills throughout his professional life
  c) The ability to assess the reliability of evidence to reach conclusions by logical deduction
  d) A continuing concern for the interests and dignity of his patients
  e) An ability to appreciate the limitations of his own knowledge, combined with a willingness when necessary to seek further help.

The latest GMC document on *Tomorrow's Doctors* sets out 14 principal recommendations, and universities throughout the United Kingdom are modifying their curriculums accordingly:

- The burden of factual information imposed on students in undergraduate medical curricula should be substantially reduced

- Learning through curiosity, the exploration of knowledge, and the critical evaluation of evidence should be promoted and should ensure a capacity for self education; the undergraduate course should be seen as the first stage in the continuum of medical education that extends throughout professional life

- Attitudes of mind and of behaviour that befit a doctor should be inculcated and should imbue a new graduate with attributes appropriate to his or her future responsibilities to patients, colleagues, and society in general

- The essential skills required by the graduate at the beginning of the preregistration year must be acquired under supervision, and proficiency in these skills must be rigorously assessed

- A "core curriculum" encompassing the essential knowledge and skills and the appropriate attitudes to be acquired at the time of graduation should be defined

- The "core curriculum" should be augmented by a series of "special study modules" which allow students to study in depth areas of particular interest to them, that provide them with the insight into scientific method and the discipline of research, and that engender an approach to medicine that is questioning and self critical

- The core curriculum should be system-based, its component parts being the combined responsibility of basic scientists and clinicians integrating their contributions to a common purpose, thus eliminating the rigid preclinical-clinical divide and the exclusive departmentally based course

- There should be emphasis throughout the course on communication skills and the other essentials of basic clinical method

- The theme of public health medicine should figure prominently in the curriculum, encompassing health promotion and illness prevention, assessment and targeting of population needs, and awareness of environmental and social factors in disease

- Clinical teaching should adapt the changing patterns in health care and should provide experience of primary care and of community medical services as well as of hospital based services

- Learning systems should be informed by modern educational theory and should draw on the wide range of technological resources available; medical schools should be prepared to share these resources to their mutual advantage

- Systems of assessment should be adapted to the new style

curriculum, encourage appropriate learning skills, and reduce emphasis on the uncritical acquisition of facts

- The design, implementation, and continued review of curricula demand the establishment of effective supervisory structures with interdisciplinary membership and adequate representation of junior staff and students

- The education committee of the GMC should ensure the implementation of its recommendations through regular reports from medical schools, continuing dialogue on the basis of informal visits, and, when necessary, by the exercise of the statutory powers given to it under the Medical Acts.

The GMC document also discusses learning systems and the methods of delivery of undergraduate courses. It notes that medical schools are well aware of the merits of learner centred, and problem orientated approaches and are striving towards their adoption, moves which the GMC strongly encourages. Most are reducing their reliance on the didactic lecture format and are

---

Box 3.2 New undergraduate curriculum

- Learner centred
- Problem orientated
- Reduction in didactic lecture
- Promotes small group learning

---

promoting small group learning wherever possible. They are seeking to improve the personal guidance available to individual students on both academic and non-academic matters: a practice which the report strongly commends.

The report also recommends certain curriculum themes, namely,

- Clinical method
- Practical skills and patient care
- Communication skills
- Human biology
- Human disease

- People in society
- The public health
- Handicap, disability, and rehabilitation
- Finding out: research and experiment.

General practice in the medical curriculum

Undergraduate medical education produces a generally educated medical graduate who has a solid foundation on which to base practical postgraduate training for whichever specialty is chosen.

The core curriculum now means that each discipline should have some part which will be relevant to all graduates regardless of their subsequent choice of specialty, and the undergraduate contribution should not attempt to teach specialised knowledge and skills. From the point of view of general practice the purpose is not to teach the undergraduates how to be general practitioners but to encourage them to learn from clinical experience in the context of general practice.

Learning in the practice is experiential and opportunistic rather than systematic, and students, with the help of tutors, should concentrate on areas which are relevant to their general undergraduate education. There is no doubt, however, that the insight which the experience gives into the work of a general practitioner may help the students to decide on their future career options. The teaching should have a structure with specific organisation. The general areas of learning should cover the context of general medical practice, how general practice integrates with self care and secondary care, and how patients go from one level to another with some knowledge of why patients seek medical advice. Secondly, the content of general medical practice should be examined and how this differs from patients seen in hospital. Thirdly, practical clinical problem solving is very important with the general practitioner demonstrating how an experienced clinician very rapidly and selectively weighs up clinical evidence and deduces the most probable cause in a particular individual patient.

Fourthly, the communication and social and professional relationships must be demonstrated. The mode of presentation is different in general practice, and communication at that level with the ability to form professional relationships are essential with the final component being integration, where knowledge and

31

Box 3.3 General areas of learning for general practice teaching

- Context of general practice
- Content of general practice
- Practical clinical problem solving
- Communication
- Social and professional relationships

---

skills derived from the various disciplines are integrated and to this is added an integrated attitude to patient care.

Time is an important factor in this teaching, and there must be some degree of protection to teachers around their normal workload. As the general practitioner is an independent contractor levels of remuneration for teaching should be appropriate to the given task. The payment for teaching under the statement of fees and allowances ended on 31 March 1996. It was recognised that this payment did not fully recognise the implications of undergraduate teaching. From 1 April 1996 payments will be made from health service budgets for the Service Increment for Teaching and Research (SIFT(R) and Additional Cost of Teaching in Scotland), and this money will be made available to departments of general practice and general practitioners who teach medical students. The exact details have still to be formulated.

During a practice attachment the student will observe how general practitioners integrate with the other members of the practice team and with other health professionals.

Most medical schools are now preparing for the latest GMC document, and there is currently great interest in the community as a resource for teaching basic clinical skills and core medicine to compensate for the increasingly specialised but diminishing teaching hospital base.

The Association for the Study of Medical Education (ASME) issued a report on community based teaching. This divided community based courses into four groups:

- Community orientated teaching in and about the community that gives students an insight into the socioeconomic environment of people who become or have been patients with the local resources available to them

- Agency based teaching, which involves a support mechanism and services available for management of illness in the community by health care providers other than general practitioners or hospital consultants

- General practice based teaching, which can be clinical teaching by using practice patients as a resource for teaching general medicine and basic clinical skills, taught by general practitioners in discussion with hospital clinicians; or a general practice attachment, which focuses on teaching general practice as a clinical specialty and is led by an academic department of general practice

- Specialist teaching in the community; clinical specialty is normally taught in hospital or taught in the community setting under the direction of the hospital specialist concerned – for example, paediatrics, psychiatry.

Within these groupings community orientated teaching can entail interviewing members of the public who may or may not be ill or, secondly, a family attachment for a prolonged period. Although this gives a wide range of options, the bulk of the teaching is general practice based.

The report noted the features of a good general practitioner attachment from the student's point of view:

- One to one teaching of the student by the general practitioner with the student sitting in on general practitioner consultations and being supervised individually for competence in history taking and performing a physical examination

- Being on call with the general practitioner and going on home visits

- Doing solo consultations with follow up briefing (or video recording if available)

- Spending time with other members of the health care team from within the practice and those working in the community, making home visits with the latter

- Promotion of self directed learning – for example, project work

- Opportunity to discuss progress with general practitioner tutor – for example, by joint completion of assessment forms or checklists of competencies

● Encouragement of reflective practice

The report notes that the main assessment of the attachment is based on the completion of worksheets. It also notes that much of the assessment is purely subjective and dependent on the personal opinion of a general practitioner tutor. With the increasing emphasis on academic audit and quality assurance this assessment is likely to become more objective.

Teacher training

Several medical schools have an active programme on teaching skills for their undergraduate medical teachers. With the likelihood of proper funding this teacher training will be the norm, and there will also be a desire to look at the quality of the teaching provided.

General practice teaching: how the organisation in clinical content differs

The students will note that the environment of general practice differs greatly from that in hospital. General practice is community based with most general practitioners working through the NHS as independent professional contractors. Each general practitioner principal has a contract with his or her health board or family health services authority to provide medical care to the named patients who are registered with him or her. This care is normally provided in association with partners and other members of the practice team.

Almost half of all doctors are general practitioners, with 33 000 in the United Kingdom. On average a doctor looks after about 1800 registered patients with the general practitioner service costing about 15% of the NHS budget, and of this 15% about one third covers staff costs and other overheads and the remainder covers the cost of prescribed drugs. On average a general practitioner conducts about 35 consultations a day in the surgery and in addition sees about three people at home. The length of a consultation varies greatly but on average is around seven minutes. The consultation is often simply one in a series of contacts building up a picture about that patient.

Population surveys have shown that most people (75%) have some complaint about their health at any given time. Only about

20% consult their general practitioner about this, and only a tiny proportion (3%) are referred on to hospital care.

Most (90%) of the problems presenting to doctors in the health service are dealt with exclusively by general practitioners, and their work must necessarily include many types and stages of illness. The general practitioner is the doctor of first contact who must be able to cope with an unlimited range of presenting symptoms. In addition to the conventional clinical skills, a

---

Box 3.4 Features of general practice

- Independent professional contractors
- Look after about 1800 registered patients
- Conducts 35 consultations a day in surgery
- Average consultation time around seven minutes
- Deal with over 90% of problems presenting in the health service
- Only 3% referred on for hospital care

---

general practitioner increasingly requires some of the skills of the educator and the manager as the emphasis changes towards promotion of health and prevention of disease and anticipatory rather than reactive management of long term disorders such as asthma and hypertension.

Summary

Undergraduate education in general practice is increasing in variety and volume. General practice is now noted to have a reputation for teaching with the postgraduate training network an ideal model to follow. There are specific topics which are best taught in a community setting and these have been highlighted.

Further reading

Fraser RC. *Clinical method in general practice.* 2nd ed. Oxford: Butterworth Heinemann, 1992.

McCrorie P, Lefford F, Perrin F. *Medical undergraduate community based teaching. A survey for ASME on current and proposed teaching in the community and in general practice in*

United Kingdom Universities. Association for the Study of Medical Education, 1993. (Occasional Publication No 3.)

Fraser RC, Preston White E. *The contribution of academic general practice to undergraduate medical education.* London: Royal College of General Practitioners, 1988. (Occasional Paper No 41.)

General Medical Council, Education Committee. *Recommendations on basic medical education.* London: GMC, 1980.

General Medical Council, Education Committee. *The teaching of behavioural sciences, community medicine and general practice in basic medical education. Report of a working party.* London: GMC, 1987.

General Medical Council. *Tomorrow's Doctors. Recommendation on undergraduate medical education.* London: GMC, 1993.

4 Vocational training for general practitioners within hospitals

Though all doctors begin their postgraduate training within hospitals, about half will eventually end up working in the community as general practitioners. Because the nature of general practice necessitates a broad training and education, covering the entire range of human disease, there is an argument that *any* training in a hospital discipline could be relevant and valuable to the aspiring general practitioner.

Common conditions occur commonly, however, and it is therefore obvious that experience in certain disciplines is more important than in others. This could be favourably compared with the new educational arrangements proposed for under-

---

Box 4.1 Hospital training and general practice

- The role of the Joint Committee on Postgraduate Training for General Practice (JCPTGP)
- The role of the postgraduate dean
- The hospital consultant as general practitioner trainer
- Role of the postgraduate tutor
- The role of the regional adviser in general practice (and course organisers)
- "Satisfactory completion" of training

---

graduates by the GMC in *Tomorrow's Doctors*, where a core curriculum of essential education is supplemented by optional modules selected by the students which best suit their own individual educational needs.

This chapter examines the roles of hospitals in the training of general practitioners under the headings listed in box 4.1.

The role of the joint committee

The vocational training regulations of 1979 decreed that "prescribed experience" should be acquired and divided hospital training into two categories. Firstly, those posts considered more important and known as "short list posts" which would be completed during one of the two years of hospital training. Secondly, other less important posts which would be completed during the other year and known as "middle year posts". These two categories are described, respectively, in boxes 4.2 and 4.3.

Box 4.2 Short list posts for medical experience for training in general practice

Six months whole time employment (or its part time equivalent) in each of two of the following specialties:

- **General medicine**
- **Geriatric medicine**
- **Paediatrics**
- **Psychiatry**
- **One of accident and emergency medicine *or* general surgery**
- **Any one of obstetrics *or* gynaecology *or* obstetrics and gynaecology**

Doctors who have carried out satisfactory training over 12 months (or its part time equivalent) in each of short list and middle year experience can apply to the joint committee, which, if satisfied, will issue a *Certificate of Prescribed Experience*. Many doctors come here from overseas, are late entrants to general practice, or are able to offer experience that does not conform strictly to the arrangements outlined in boxes 4.2 and 4.3. Under

---

Box 4.3 Middle year posts for medical experience for training in general practice

Any "educationally approved post" which is approved for the purposes of training in a hospital specialty or in the specialty of community medicine (now known as public health medicine) by the royal college or faculty for that specialty *and* selected by a regional postgraduate medical education committee for the purposes of training for the provision of general medical services

---

the regulations they are still able to offer experience they feel to be equivalent for consideration by the joint committee, which can, if satisfied, issue a *Certificate of Equivalent Experience* that has equal force.

Of course, before the doctors receive their "certificate of satisfactory completion of training" from the joint committee they must also undertake satisfactorily 12 months' full time employment (or its part time equivalent) as a trainee general practitioner, and this phase of training is described in another chapter.

At the end of "satisfactory completion" of each phase of hospital training doctors should receive a VTR 2 certificate from their hospital trainer which, along with a VTR 1 certificate from their general practitioner trainer, should be submitted to the joint committee as evidence of their experience. In normal circumstances these various certificates, with each trainer's signature authenticated by a countersignature from the regional adviser, will be sufficient evidence for the joint committee to issue a certificate of prescribed or equivalent experience. No doctor can become a general practitioner principal on an NHS health authority list without such a certificate. (Special rules apply for those doctors who were already on a medical list before 15 February 1981.)

The postgraduate dean

Postgraduate deans have important responsibilities over the whole range of postgraduate medical education as outlined in chapter 2. Not least of these is their responsibility for the education and training of general practitioners, usually mediated through regional advisers in general practice.

Hospitals, of course, are institutions primarily concerned with service to patients rather than with the education of doctors, and this also holds for the teaching hospitals which have additional responsibilities for both undergraduate and postgraduate medical education. The main duty of the postgraduate dean and the regional adviser is to ensure that there is in place a proper balance between the service duties of doctors and their education.

All hospital doctors except for consultants, associate specialists, and clinical assistants are in the "training grades". Unfortunately, there are still those managements in some hospitals which are so short sighted as to forget the fact that such doctors in training are the seed of the future and that properly structured training and medical education are as much for the benefit of the NHS and of good patient care as they are for the benefit of the individual doctor.

Doctors in the preregistration year immediately after graduation have their education monitored by the universities and the GMC. More senior doctors, in the career registrar and specialist registrar grades, have special attention paid to their needs by the various specialist colleges and the postgraduate deans. Unfortunately, most training for general practice takes place in that grade in the middle, the senior house officer grade, where there is least educational supervision. This grade has been graphically described in the past as "the lost tribe" of medical education.

Those senior house officers in training for general practice, therefore, are senior enough to be a "useful pair of hands" but often too junior to attract the attention of their consultant teachers as aspiring specialists. Among consultants there are, of course, notable exceptions, but the postgraduate deans must act as junior doctors' advocates in the protection of their educational interests.

The hospital consultant as an educator of general practitioners

All consultants have a professional and ethical duty to instruct their juniors in the special skills they themselves have acquired. Unfortunately, two factors often militate against success in this sphere with regard to general practice. Firstly, unlike general practitioner trainers, few consultants undergo any special instruction in *how* to teach. Within general practice itself many new techniques have developed that have actively moved away from the didactic lecture. These techniques include small group teaching, role play and simulated clinical encounters, the use of videorecording as a teaching tool, and a problem solving approach to education – all of which require some teaching of the teacher.

The second problem area concerns *what* is taught. The average hospital consultant is not excited by the routine or mundane case and most presentations of hospital cases tend to concentrate on the unusual or rare condition. What is forgotten, to the detriment of the general practitioner trainee, is that the spectrum of presentations within a hospital specialty is totally at odds with what presents within the community. What is humdrum in a hospital is in itself unusual in any typical general practice. What general practitioner trainees need, therefore, is thorough and systematic instruction in those cases that conceivably might present occasionally in a normal general practice and which would need accurate diagnosis and referral within an appropriate time scale.

Hospital consultant trainers are, however, improving year on year, and the suggestion contained in the report of the Calman subgroup on general practice (1995) that all training for a hospital specialty should have the opportunity to spend an elective period within general practice should lead to even better performance as general practitioner educators.

The postgraduate tutor

Postgraduate deans are officers with large geographical areas to monitor, and their local representatives in the various hospitals are the postgraduate tutors. The terms of reference for postgraduate tutors are described in chapter 2, but they also have a special responsibility towards general practitioner trainees in hospital. They run postgraduate centres within hospitals and are in immediate charge of devolved educational budgets from the deans. The postgraduate centre and its attached medical library is an important focus for postgraduate training, and the tutors should be stimulating and coordinating all educational activity within the hospital setting.

Most specialists will arrange clinical meetings within their own narrow specialties, but postgraduate tutors must ensure that all training grade doctors, but particularly general practitioner trainees, have a leavening of educational input that is outside their own specialist area of interest at the time.

The regional inspections by the joint committee ensure that all those in the training grades who have committed themselves as eventual general practitioners will be able to attend a half day release course that attempts to bring a general practice perspective to the experience that is gained within the hospital job. As postgraduate tutors are almost invariably hospital consultants themselves, it is important that they involve the regional advisers in general practice, but more usually the regional advisers' local officers, and the course organisers (associate advisers in Scotland).

The regional adviser in general practice

The Regional Advisers in General Practice supervise the educational approval for the hospital posts within their region which are used in general practice training. The overall responsibility is with the Postgraduate Dean but this is normally devolved to the Regional Adviser when doctors are training for general practice. The educational content of the post must be satisfactory and the feedback from the Course Organiser is an important link in the information chain.

In England and Wales the approval is normally carried out by the respective Royal College and in Scotland by the Regional Postgraduate Committee. In addition to the approval process the Course Organisers normally arrange a programme of education for the doctors training for general practice who are in their hospital component.

"Satisfactory completion"

In the past it was thought that mere attendance for work within the various components of training was sufficient to merit the award of a VTR 2 (the necessary "ticket" for the certification process). In response to evidence that some training was poor in quality, however, the meaning of satisfactory completion of training was codified in August 1990 by a joint letter from the chairman of the GMSC, the chairman of the joint committee, and the chairman of council of the royal college. This letter defined "satisfactory completion" as indicating "a satisfactory level of competence, in the assessment of the person signing, in the field of medicine to which the statement relates". Given this definition, it is now implicit that whoever signs the certificate must have some method of assessing that competence.

Assessment can be of two types: *formative* or *summative* – that is, educational or regulatory. These concepts are explored further in a later chapter, but it is now a minimum requirement of the joint committee that formative or educational assessment must be an integral part of all general practice training, and this applies equally to that part of training undertaken within hospitals. Therefore, not only must the hospital training post contain sufficient education relevant to general practice, the application of that education must now be assessed before the experience is certified as having been completed satisfactorily – that is, the trainee has acquired a degree of competence.

Training curriculum

One of the main current areas of concern for educators of general practitioners is the content of the education which is imparted to GP registrars while in the hospital component. This is compounded by the fact that many registrars undertaking such posts are "undeclared" aspiring family doctors. This can be for two reasons; firstly, that they may not yet have decided on their final career path, but also, secondly, that there is a perception that the quality of training and access to study leave is often second rate if the young doctor declares such an intention.

A "core curriculum" for general practice implies that hospital training should cover only that core and should have a slant towards the presentation of disease within a community; it also implies that such doctors should not be used merely as "a pair of hands" to satisfy service demands. Training for general practice demands that a proper curriculum is defined and addressed, that there is easy access to half day release programmes, and that those leaving such hospital posts are equipped to undertake general practice with relevant knowledge and skills. There must also be a strategy to train GP registrars in the elements of the "minor specialties" (such as ophthalmology and ear, nose, and throat) without having to undertake a full six month post.

Further reading

General Medical Council. *Tomorrow's Doctors*. London: GMC, 1993.

Joint Committee on Postgraduate Teaching for General Practice. *National Health Service vocational training for general practice: a guide to certification*. London: JCPTGP, 1995.

Joint Committee on Postgraduate Training for General Practice. *Accreditation of regions and schemes for vocational training in general practice: general guidance.* London: JCPTGP, 1990.

Joint Committee on Postgraduate Training for General Practice. *Selection of posts in hospital and community medicine for vocational training in general practice.* London: JCPTGP, 1980.

National Association of Health Authorities and Trusts. *Partners in learning: developing postgraduate training and continuing education for general practice.* London: NAHAT, 1994.

Department of Health. *Hospital doctors: training for the future: the report of the working group on specialist medical training.* Manchester: Health Publications Unit, 1993.

Department of Health. *Hospital doctors: training for the future: a supplementary report by the working group commissioned to consider the implications for general medical practice arising from the principal report.* Manchester: Health Publications Unit, 1995.

5 Vocational training: the practice component, structure, methods, and deficiencies

The in practice year adds the vocational element to the general professional training undertaken in hospital. The overall aim of the practice year is to acquire the basic general practice competencies and lay a sound foundation for further professional development. To achieve these aims a practice should provide the general practitioner registrar with sheltered working conditions in which he or she has time and opportunity to explore the range of general practice. This should provide:

- Space for professional growth

- Challenge to keep the registrar sufficiently stretched and intellectually stimulated

- Encouragement to respond to patients in whole person terms

- A model from which to discover his or her own professional identity.

As general practice continues to undergo great change it is important to produce doctors who are thinking, responsive, and responsible and who can adapt to new situations. The practical nature of general practice demands that much of the instruction is through doing, and adequate backup should be available at all times so that potential learning experiences can be maximised.

This can happen only when the practice is prepared for training with all the partners playing a part.

To conform to the requirements of the Joint Committee on Postgraduate Training for General Practitioners, doctors training for general practice either undergo a recognised three year vocational training scheme or are responsible for making up their scheme, which entails obtaining the appropriate hospital posts and then a year as a general practitioner registrar in general practice. The process of selection of a GP registrar post in the self construct scheme should entail an input from without the practice in advising potential GP registrars as to the requirements for the completion of their training. Those who are on a set scheme are much more likely to have supervision from the general practice education network during their hospital component. It is important, however, that only those who are of a satisfactory standard should progress to their year in general practice. If there are obvious deficiencies in their training then further hospital training would be advisable before undertaking the GP registrar year.

Appointment of trainers and training practices

All regions have their own criteria for the appointment of their trainers and training practices. Minimal criteria are set by the joint committee and all regions must reach those criteria. The personal qualities of trainers are important. They should be enthusiastic, competent and caring general practitioners working in well organised practices. They should have a desire to teach with time to do so, with positive attitudes towards training from their partners and practice team; the practice should also demonstrate clinical competence and quality measures in their care of patients. The trainers should be aware of current educational methods, and the practice organisation and premises must be geared for training.

The training practice: organisation and management

The practice must prepare to have the GP registrar as an integrated member of the practice team. This entails a gentle introduction to the practice with an increasing workload and in the latter parts of the training year functioning as a partner. This is essential in preparation for independent practice. The registrar will learn a great deal from contact on a day to day basis with members of the practice team, but this should be supplemented by teaching involving these members of staff. In an ideal world general practitioner registrars should have consulting rooms of their own, but if this is not possible then space must always be available for the various consulting and training activities. The workload of the practice should allow the registrar teaching to be integrated with the normal running of the practice. All partners and staff should be supportive of training as this is now regarded as a practice commitment. The patients should also be informed in the practice leaflet as to the high priority given to training and also their important role in the development of the training process. The use of video for training purposes should also be explained with their rights regarding participating in this training.

Box 5.1 Organisation of training practice for training

- GP registrar an integrated member
- Day to day contact with all members of the practice team
- Teaching integrated with normal running of the practice
- Teaching is a practice commitment

The trainer as an employer

The general practitioner registrar must have a contract of employment, with the trainer being aware of his or her obligation as an employer and assisting the registrar with all entitlements under the statement of fees and allowances. The standard BMA contract is the one normally used.

Ability to make available the necessary time for teaching

This is by good organisation, and at the time of an accreditation visit trainers should be able to demonstrate the value of a well run appointment system or other methods of access flexible enough to allow patients to be seen immediately when necessary. They should be able to demonstrate effective arrangements within the practice for home visiting and for services such as health promotion, chronic disease management, maternity, family planning, and child health surveillance.

The practice should have policies for home visiting, continuity of care, and emergency care. The GP registrar should obtain first hand experience of effective organisation, practice management, and financial matters in a general practice. The practice should demonstrate a system of management so that the registrar can learn through experience. Workload is a particularly important factor, and when this is considered there has to be a balance between ensuring that on the one hand the practice can give adequate time to its teaching commitments and on the other it can provide sufficient clinical experience comparable with that expected in an average general practice.

At the time of a visit there should be effective use of the practice team in patient care; the premises should be adequate for the number of patients served, and there should be a sufficient number of consulting rooms so that the GP registrar is able to consult during the same surgery sessions as the trainer or other partners. There should be an efficient records system. Practice records must have clinical notes, letters, and the results of investigations filed in chronological order. Long term drug treatment should be clearly discernible in the records, and important past events should be summarised.

Effective organisation, practice management, and financial control are very important in modern general practice, and it is essential for GP registrars to acquire skills and obtain first hand experience in these areas. It is important that a practice provides teaching on the business aspects of general practice, the principles of management, communication within the primary care team, business methods, medical budgeting, and practice accounts. Such teaching should also cover economic aspects of health care illustrated by the practice policies – for example, in achieving cost-effectiveness in prescribing and the use of health

---

Box 5.2 Important service areas for GP registrars

- Effective organisation within practice
- Practice management
- Financial control
- Health care delivery

services resources. Fundholding and locality purchasing are also important issues.

The use of the hospital services with the interaction between primary and secondary care are also important areas to be covered during the GP registrar year.

Quality issues

The practice should be concerned in setting standards, with the GP registrar taking a part in this with regular experience of determining and reviewing criteria and standards of care. This also entails performance monitoring within the practice and thus acquiring the knowledge and skills needed to carry out and implement the results of practice audit. In preparing for the future the registrar will be responsible for the care of individual patients, care of groups of patients, the practice population and the practice and health care team and also involved with the community and the wider profession.

The trainer as teacher

Before employing a first GP registrar trainers will have attended a basic residential trainers' course which will cover their role as teachers. They will also be expected to attend their local trainers groups with further attendance at courses to develop teaching skills and methods of training. The personal qualities of trainers are very important as their example will provide the registrar with the appropriate role model. Trainers must have an enthusiasm and keenness to teach as well as an ability to motivate a registrar. Trainers must also be willing to monitor the progress of their teaching and to discuss this regularly with the GP registrars and their peers. Past teaching experience with other groups – for example, medical students – will be considered important in their preparation.

Attendance at courses help trainers understand the processes of learning and teaching and provide opportunity to explore their teaching responsibilities with their peers in trainer groups and to appreciate the wide range of local resources that can contribute to their teaching task. The organisation of teaching is very important and the trainer should ascertain the GP registrar's needs. At the beginning of the year the registrar's strengths and areas of need should be identified. The year's teaching should be geared towards building on the strengths and meeting the learning needs. Progress on achieving these targets should be reviewed on a regular basis and appropriate action taken. This is one of the reasons for formative assessment. Tutorials should take place at least once a week in protected time and should last for at least one hour. The topic should be planned jointly in advance. The registrar should be given specific preparation tasks, and the trainer should also prepare for tutorials. There should be regular planned feedback sessions for the registrar to comment on the teaching programme. In addition, all members of the practice should take the opportunity to engage in informal teaching whenever the opportunity should arise.

Box 5.3 The trainer as teacher

- **Attends basic trainers' course**
- **Can identify the GP registrar needs**
- **Continues to develop teaching skills**

Teaching abilities

The trainer should have a clear idea of what is to be achieved, the ability to identify a registrar's needs, and an understanding of how these can be met. The trainer must continue to develop teaching skills. These would be related mainly to one to one teaching, involvement in group teaching, the ability to give feedback by recognising the teaching potential in everyday events in general practice, development of a style which is discussive and allows the GP registrar's potential to be reached. This would be GP registrar centred and would be unique for that particular registrar. It is important that the trainer analyses the various components of everyday tasks and passes these on to the registrar. Everyday work and the backup of evidence are powerful influences on the learning process. Involvement in the planning and delivery of the content of the teaching year are important aspects of ownership.

Formative assessment

Formative assessment is educational and should be free of threat. Its main aim is to allow strengths and weaknesses to be recognised and also to give feedback on knowledge and performance. Trainers have always assessed GP registrars without necessarily using the term assessment. Case discussion over coffee, performance at tutorials, casual feedback from partners, staff, and patients all contribute to the "gut feeling" which trainers develop about an individual registrar. The advantage of this kind of assessment is that it is continuous, natural, and unthreatening. It also requires minimum time and effort. The disadvantage of this kind of assessment is that it is often subliminal and random with no record of the areas covered. It can lead to a cosy, supportive, and unchallenging relationship. In addition, the impressions gained are wholly subjective. Therefore, although continuous informal assessment is desirable, it must be supplemented with a balanced programme of structured assessment.

Formal assessment can seem threatening both to trainers and GP registrars. It should be borne in mind, however, that the assessment is being carried out for educational reasons and that the emphasis is on formative assessment. In the context of general practice training we need assessment to answer the following questions:

- What does the GP registrar already know?

- What does the GP registrar need to know?

- Is the GP registrar making satisfactory progress?

- Has our teaching been successful?

No single assessment method is capable of providing the information necessary for useful formative assessment. The range of methods recommended should provide reliable, valid, and useful data.

Checklist – The checklist is designed to assess the GP registrar's confidence in dealing with particular situations. Used regularly it will indicate topics in which the registrar feels more help is required and also those in which the registrar feels completely confident. Although confidence and competence are not the same thing, there is a useful correlation between the two. The checklist can be specifically used in tutorial planning to make sure that no significant gaps are left.

Video assessment – Joint observation of consultations is the only method by which the clinical work of the registrar can be directly monitored. Many methods such as sitting in and audio taping have been used in the past. Video recording provides the least disruptive and most effective method. It is appreciated that video teaching is threatening to the GP registrar and if badly handled can be destructive. For this reason trainers are encouraged to use a specific course on teaching in the consultation by using the method pioneered by Pendleton *et al* (*The Consultation*). Fear of the video decreases with repeated use.

Interview with course organiser – This will be used simply to check that the GP registrar is settling well into the practice and has no specific problems.

Manchester rating – This set of rating scales was devised several years ago and should enable the trainer to attempt to make an assessment of the general practitioner registrar's performance in a variety of areas – for example, problem solving, clinical judgment, and professional attitudes. The registrar should also complete the scale thus enabling a mutually agreed assessment of the registrar's performance.

Multiple choice question – This is a measurement of factual knowledge and should enable both trainer and GP registrar to detect relevant gaps in the knowledge base. This is normally arranged at a regional level so that the registrars can see how they stand in relation to their peers.

An objective structured clinical examination (OSCE) – This assessment tool is designed to present the registrar with a standardised clinical problem to deal with. Each question has a predetermined marking schedule so should be objective. This

---

Box 5.4 Formative assessment

- **Checklist**
- **Video assessment**
- **Interview with course organiser**
- **Manchester rating**
- **Multiple choice question**
- **Objective structured clinical examination (OSCE)**

technique is used for assessing practical skills but can also be used to look at decision making and attitudes.

Annual feedback

In addition, the end of year reports by the GP registrar can be used during formative assessment. This has a statement as to what should happen regarding practice structure: in organisation, patient records, appointment systems and home visits, library facilities, information technology, audit, terms and conditions of employment, practice management, premises and equipment, and the primary health care team.

In relation to experience the introductory period, clinical experience, out of hours experience, paediatric surveillance, minor surgery and hospital clinics are all covered. Supervision is dealt with both in surgery and out of hours. Case discussion and teaching looks at the GP registrar's needs: tutorials, review and feedback, assessment, informal teaching, project work and research, and educational day release are all dealt with. In addition, the overall practice ethos is covered. The basis of this report is what should happen during the training year and can be an excellent formative tool for receiving feedback during the year.

The trainer/GP registrar relationship is based on the adult learning principle with both actively concerned in the learning process. All registrars are individuals and their needs and personalities must be clearly understood. In addition, trainers should be aware of their personal and educational shortcomings and personalities should not affect this special relationship. An effective trainer/GP registrar relationship needs self awareness, honesty and openness, mutual respect, sharing each other's values and goals, and being useful to each other.

Box 5.5 Adult learning

- Active involvement in learning process
- Individual learning needs identified
- Look at outcomes to see if achieved

Other teaching

All registrars will have a structured programme outside the practice at their half day release when they meet other registrars.

Increasingly this is becoming GP registrar centred with the registrars being responsible for their own learning process. In addition, special tuition is given in areas of importance – for example, child health surveillance, minor surgery, information technology, time management, and preparation for the MRCGP.

Difficulties with trainer/GP registrar relationship

It is unusual to have such a problem as the trainer normally chooses the registrar after interview and taking up references following guidelines set by the region. If, however, there is any difficulty between the trainer and the registrar then advice would first be given by the course organiser, and if the problem is unlikely to resolve the regional adviser would become involved with the question of moving the registrar to another practice becoming a distinct possibility.

Deficiencies

The main deficiencies are as a result of the day to day pressures of general practice when less time and commitment is given to training that would be ideal. The stresses and demands of the 1990 contract and the subsequent demands of general practice have added to this process. Feedback from registrars suggests that the areas where there are deficiencies are audit, formative assessment, the management structure within general practice, and the business aspects of general practice. Registrars admit that they are less interested in the service aspects of practice, and this undoubtedly could have an influence in this deficiency.

Further reading

Havelock P, Hasler J, Flew R, *et al. Professional education for general practice.* Oxford: Oxford General Practice Series, 1995.

Pendleton D, *et al. The consultation.* Oxford: Oxford University Press, 1984.

Newble D, Cannon R. *A handbook for medical teachers.* 3rd ed. Lancaster: Kluwer Academic, 1994.

Joint Committee on Postgraduate Training for General Practice. *Training for general practice.* London: JCPTGP, 1982.

Joint Committee on Postgraduate Training for General Practice. *Accreditation of regions and schemes for vocational training in general practice.* London: JCPTGP, 1992.

Joint Committee on Postgraduate Training for General Practice. *Recommendations to regions for the establishment of criteria for the approval and reapproval of trainers in general practice.* London: JCPTGP, 1993.

6 The training practice: section 63 funding

Although a trainer is appointed with the prime responsibility for training, it is now recognised that training is a practice commitment and should concern all partners in varying degrees, both in the formal and informal teaching. The training practice should provide an appropriate environment for learning. During their early months in the practice the GP registrars will receive much supervision and protection, but this will lessen as the year progresses. A great deal of what the GP registrar learns will be from modelling, and it is important that training practices provide the highest level of patient care with appropriate organisation. This will reinforce for the registrars what can be done in the day to day management of patients and also help to prepare them for their time as independent practitioners. Within the training practice there is a vast amount of skill and the GP registrar should be exposed to all aspects of this.

The library

It is important that training practices have good libraries with up to date books and a collection of current journals. Most regions have a list of core books which can be referred to. With the move to evidence based medicine a number of practice libraries are also subscribing to Medline (see chapter 14). There should also be books relating to the other health professions within the practice.

Clinical records

Well organised practice records allow the GP registrar to be aware of past information at the beginning of a consultation.

Records should be maintained for all doctor-patient contacts. There should be a clear and effective system for the creation and updating of summaries, and there should be a written statement about the content which should include preventive data. Records also provide the basis of teaching for audit and for research projects. The development of preventive medicine and health promotion in a practice partially depends on its ability to identify patients by age and sex, by morbidity, and by the factors which place certain groups at risk. Many practices have developed systems to help the GP registrars review their work. These include age-sex registers, disease index, and personal logs. Much of this information is now available on computer.

Computers

Computerisation within general practice has been spectacular, and the practice should be able to demonstrate basic skills in the use of information technology to the GP registrar. Some doctors now have desk top computers, and, in addition to providing a basic age-sex register and carrying out repeat prescribing, computers have a tremendous potential to help in the improvement of clinical care. One of their most valuable functions is the identification of groups and subgroups of patients – for example, patients with hypertension – with specific prompts to encourage screening.

The partners

It is important that all the partners are integrated towards the training process within the practice. Each should give teaching in their recognised topics of strength and should be available to help the GP registrar on an informal basis. As the registrars are in a learning situation they should be involved in all practice meetings both with other members of the primary care team and business meetings involving the partners themselves. It is also important that the partners recognise that they must provide protected time for the partner involved in the training process. This will normally be the trainer, who will take a reduced commitment of other work to fulfil teaching duties.

The practice team

The registrar has a great deal to learn from receptionists, secretaries, the practice manager, practice nurses, district nurses, health visitors, and social workers in addition to some other health professionals. They should be integrated into the work of the practice and also have an input into the GP registrar's teaching programme. This tends to occur on an informal basis, but there is a case for this being more formal. All should be involved in the delivery of health care, the development of the management of chronic diseases, and further development of protocols within the practice; these activities would provide the necessary ownership of the material as a practice.

Workload

This must be sufficient to provide the GP registrars with adequate experience as all teaching has to be placed in context. They also must receive enough experience so that they can deal with the real world of general practice when they finish the registrar year. Their early consultations should be at 20 minute intervals, moving fairly quickly to 15 minutes, and, as soon as they are able, to 10 minute appointments. In the latter parts of training there should be some opportunity for consulting at a more rapid pace so that the registrar is aware of the variations within general practice. Workload should be sufficient to give the registrar experience but should not be too great so that inadequate time is available for teaching.

Relationship with other health professionals and hospital

This will tend to vary from practice to practice, and a resource booklet giving the GP registrars guidelines is extremely useful.

Audit and quality assurance

The trainer and other members of the practice team should be actively involved in audit and should be able to demonstrate this to a GP registrar. It is important in this work that all members of the practice are involved and that standards and criteria are set with individual responsibilities defined. This provides the partnership with ownership and a higher likelihood of a positive involvement and outcome.

Patients

Patients will be aware from a long attachment to the practice and also from the practice leaflet that the practice is involved in the training process. This could lead to situations where trainer and GP registrar are present at consultations and also occasions when the patient's permission is sought for the use of video. It is important to convey to patients that they can refuse to be videoed and that this will not affect the service given.

Box 6.1 Features of training practice

- The library
- Clinical records
- Computers
- The partners
- The practice team
- Workload
- Relationship with other professionals and hospital
- Audit and quality assurance
- Patients

Section 63 funding

The first publicly funded scheme for further education in general practice was based on section 48 of the NHS Act 1946, and general practice was the only branch of medicine provided for in this way. The Department of Health (then the Ministry of Health) made universities with medical schools responsible for approving courses in their regions. This responsibility was exercised by postgraduate deans, who were in turn accountable to the university postgraduate committees. This funding was replaced by section 63 of the Health Service and Public Health Act 1968, which provided for the funding of further education and vocational training for general practitioners. The approval of activities under section 63 was fully delegated by the Department of Health and Social Security (DHSS) to the postgraduate deans, and only they could decide whether a course was suitable for approval. Approval of a course meant that general practitioners who attended were authorised to claim a locum allowance and travel and subsistence. Allowances for locums were withdrawn in 1966, when the review body included an element in the basic practice allowance to cover this cost.

From 1966 until 1977 seniority allowances, which were introduced in the family doctors' charter negotiations, were payable only if a general practitioner had attended the requisite number of educational sessions. This link between an element of remuneration and recorded attendances at section 63 courses was strongly opposed by the profession for many years. The government agreed to end it only after cash limits were applied to the funding of section 63 in 1976. Until that time the expenditure on section 63 courses and expenses had been open ended. In 1976 zero rating was introduced, which meant that no central costs were incurred for courses but the general practitioner could claim travel and subsistence expenses. The introduction of compulsory vocational training in 1981 meant that the cost of training would also be met from section 63. This led, in England, to cash limits being imposed on the travel and subsistence budget.

Wood *et al* (1980) looked at section 63 activities and considered that continuing education for general practice was not given the attention that it deserved. The growth in section 63 was noted, and the number of recorded attendances between 1969 and 1977 had risen by 108%. The authors thought that this suggested that the decision to make the payment of seniority allowances conditional on a minimum of 12 hours attendance at section 63 activities each year had had a positive influence on attendance though not necessarily, of course, on learning. It was noted at this time that although the number of activities had increased greatly, the characteristics of the meetings had not.

The link to seniority payments ceased in 1977, and with the introduction of the 1990 contract and the postgraduate education allowance section 63 was then only responsible for the budget related to training. This is now given as a total budget to

---

Box 6.2 Section 63

- Only related to training
- Provides funding for course fees
- Provides funding for travel and subsistence
- Small group teaching is usual format

---

postgraduate deans with the budgets managed by the regional advisers. Within the budget there is funding for course fees and also funding for travel and subsistence. This provides the infrastructure for all the training activity which takes place outside the practices. It also allows for residential courses, where a lot of important exchange in learning takes place. With the movement to small group teaching this format is a very important part of training courses.

Further reading

Joint Committee on Postgraduate Training for General Practice. *Recommendations to regions for the establishment of criteria for the approval and reapproval of trainers in general practice*. London: JCPTGP, 1993.

Ellis N. *What is happening to section 63? BMJ* 1985; **290**: 1527–30.

Wood J, Byrne PS. *Section 63 activities*. London: Royal College of General Practitioners, 1980. (Occasional Paper No 11.)

Branthwaite A, Ross A, Henshaw A, *et al. Continuing education for general practitioners*. London: Royal College of General Practitioners, 1988. (Occasional Paper No 38.)

7 Vocational training: completion, accreditation, and summative assessment

Accreditation is individual and signifies that the person has reached the appropriate standard. Within a profession the members have specialised knowledge and skills, and accreditation is the statement that allows the doctor to work independently.

The Joint Committee on Postgraduate Training for General Practice is an autonomous body formed in 1975. It is composed of representatives of the profession and includes two general practitioner registrars. It is the body prescribed under the vocational training regulations as responsible for issuing certificates to doctors who have satisfied it that they are entitled to them. The vocational training regulations were amended in December 1994 with the joint committee being granted the responsibility for the supervision of vocational training particularly the assessment of training. At that time the joint committee was formally designated as the competent authority for vocational training. When granted the certificate is valid indefinitely and may be used whenever the doctor wants to apply to become a principal in general practice in the NHS. The joint committee is also described in chapter 4.

Until 1990 the regulations explained what a trainee had to do before becoming a general practitioner principal. This did not include the necessity for any formal assessment as trainers (VTR/1 certificate), and consultants (VTR/2 certificate) had only

Box 7.1 Joint Committee on Postgraduate Training for General Practice

- Responsible for issuing certificates to doctors who have satisfactorily completed training
- Responsibility for the supervision of vocational training
- Competent authority for vocational training

to sign a form saying that the trainee had satisfactorily completed the post. No one until recently had defined what satisfactory completion actually meant.

Within the current regulations the experience required to obtain a certificate is of two types. Firstly, prescribed experience as set out in the regulations is fairly straightforward and applies to nearly all trainees. This is normally two years in hospital and one year as a GP registrar. Equivalent experience is experience not usually of the standard pattern but is recognised as being equal to prescribed experience. For prescribed experience a registrar merely obtains statements of satisfactory completion for each post and sends them to the joint committee, who then send the registrar a certificate. The joint committee will issue certificates "if satisfied" that the doctor has satisfactorily completed vocational training. The number of alternatives is large but of the two year period in hospital at least two of the six month posts, and preferably three, have to be from the following shortlist of six specialties:

- Accident and emergency or general surgery
- General medicine
- Geriatric medicine
- Obstetrics or gynaecology, or both
- Paediatrics
- Psychiatry.

At the present moment regional advisers encourage those training for practice to carry out their four components from this list and then to have their period of one year in general practice. There are various combinations of when the general practice component takes place but increasingly the final period of training is in general practice.

Box 7.2 Vocational training prescribed experience

- Normally two years in hospital and one year as a general practitioner registrar
- Six month posts from shortlist specialty and one year as general practitioner registrar

---

Summative assessment

Summative assessment or regulatory accreditation is when decisions are made about a doctor's future, and in this process every effort must be made to devise fair tests so that decisions are correct and based on appropriate criteria – that is, reliable and valid. Those undertaking the test should be informed of these criteria and the methods used, and if possible this information should be given at the beginning of a course. In general practice an effective system of summative assessment is essential: firstly, because of the need for objective evidence of competence for the individual GP registrar; secondly, the need for objective evidence of competence to deal with the current anxieties expressed by the public, the health departments, and the wider profession; and, thirdly, the need for demonstration of quality in standards of training.

Box 7.3 Why summative assessment

- Need for objective evidence of competence
- Protect and reassure the public
- Demonstration of quality in standards of training

Competence is used loosely, and it is important to separate competence from performance. Clinical competence is what the doctor can do, and performance is defined as what the doctor actually does in real clinical practice. It is easier to assess competence than performance, and competence does not always correlate highly with performance in practice. In the postgraduate field, however, closer attention is given to assessing performance. When an assessment tool is developed it is important to consider the important criteria of validity, reliability, and feasibility.

The establishment of validity is the first priority, and this means ensuring that the assessment measures what it is supposed to measure. The content must be appropriate to what is being tested, and without this all the other attributes become less important. The framework should be provided across several dimensions of testing to increase the validity.

A valid assessment looks at areas of competence which are important, the criteria used are relevant, and the testing process does not in itself have an effect on performance. There are several subspecies of validity:

- Content validity – the assessment looks at areas relevant to the skills being assessed in sufficient breadth and depth
- Face validity – the method and the areas assessed look appropriate
- Predictive validity – the assessment predicts accurately the ability to perform adequately in the prospective professional role. Predictive validity is almost impossible to measure because of the multiple confounding influences which affect doctors' performance after certification. It also takes a long time for data on long term performance to emerge.

Reliability is the expression of consistency and precision of the test measurement with the feasibility being related to the practicality of applying the test within the resources available. When all of these are considered in relation to the knowledge, skills, and attitudes required by the practising general practitioner then the test must have a high degree of resemblance to what the general practitioner does in daily work.

In the testing of general practitioners and other specialists, achievement of minimal standards of competence is what is important. As this is the main purpose of assessment then a criterion referenced approach is the most appropriate – that is, that the tasks can be completed by minimally competent general practitioners. This approach necessitates the determination of the standard before the examination is conducted rather than to wait to see the overall results before doing so. It is extremely difficult to do but everyone concerned with the assessment is forced to consider each item and ask themselves if it is relevant and set at an appropriate level of difficulty.

Development of summative assessment

A joint committee report on assessment in 1987 concluded that the current approach to assessment for certification under the NHS vocational training regulations had been examined and found wanting. It stated that assessment, both for educational and standard setting purposes, was an underdeveloped aspect of vocational training. It recommended that summative assessment should be given a higher profile and in particular said that training for general practice, including assessment, should reflect the content of the clinical services for patients more clearly. The joint committee would be responsible through its operation of the NHS vocational training regulations for ensuring a minimal standard of competence of doctors completing training, and statements of satisfactory completion of training should therefore represent the actual performance of a general practitioner registrar rather than indicate attendance at a training programme.

A letter in August 1990 from the chairmen of the joint committee, the royal college, and the GMSC stated that the three bodies were concerned with the standards in general practice regarding satisfactory completion and indicated that this meant satisfactory competence in the assessment of the person. This would affect both posts in hospital and general practice. The letter concluded that this statement assured the public that doctors completing vocational training achieved a satisfactory standard of competence and performance. During 1991 an important decision of the joint committee was to agree the need for a national standard of entry into general practice. At its meeting on 22 August the following resolution was proposed, seconded and carried by a majority vote.

> "This committee accepts the need for a national standard of entry into general practice and therefore the necessity to apply a system of assessment which is credible both to the public and the profession".

Consequently the main thrust of the committee's work has been in the development of its policy in assessment, to identify nationally acceptable indicators, to measure progress and clinical competence and to link satisfactory completion of vocational training in general practice to the agreed attributes for independent practice. A working party on assessment was given the task of exploring, as a matter of urgency, the practical implications of the introduction of a national standard of entry into general practice and the system of assessment which will be necessary to carry it out. At the time of the interim report in May 1992 there was a unanimous support for a uniform national standard of entry to general practice.

The report of the summative assessment working party was adopted by the joint committee at its meeting on 27 May 1993. The joint committee suggested that summative assessment be implemented from 1 January 1996 (later changed to 1996-7). They noted that a more objective process of assessment will be necessary to ensure a minimum standard of competence of all doctors entering the discipline of general practice. The assessment should take place both within the hospital posts and within general practice. They recommended that any system of summative (that is, regulatory) assessment should contain four elements:

- Tests of factual knowledge and problem solving

- Submission of practical work

- Evaluation of clinical and consulting skills

- The trainer's overall assessment.

The joint committee thought it important that a truly national standard was developed and that any summative assessment process should entail scrutiny from without the region and that external assessors should be involved. Additionally, a region's system of summative assessment would be reviewed by the joint committee as part of its regular visits. The joint committee package will still have the trainer's signature as the final part of the process, but this signature will now be informed by an external process. The previous single informed signature had a low consumption of resources but was condemned for its lack of validity, reliability, discrimination, and neutrality. The number of trainees who did not receive a certificate under these regulations was very small.

In the GMSC survey of all general practitioners, of 24 779 who responded to the question, "Did the vocational training certificate issued by the JCPTGP provide sufficient proof of a GP trainee's competence to practice as a general practitioner?" only half agreed or strongly agreed with that statement, demonstrating the unhappiness about the system existing at that time.

The royal college had highlighted as a problem the methods for determining the competence of a doctor on completing vocational training in 1985. In their 1994 policy document the college stated that doctors in completing training should demonstrate their competence for independent practice through an objective assessment that operates to a national standard. In July 1993 the royal college reiterated its view on the need for an objective assessment of the competence of doctors on the completion of vocational training. This view was endorsed by the National Association of Health Authorities and Trusts (NAHAT) in March 1994. They stated that such a system is needed to reassure patients, colleagues in other disciplines, health authorities, and the government that new recruits to NHS general practice have demonstrated their competence to practice independently to a national standard.

Summative assessment in west of Scotland

To develop summative assessment within the west of Scotland a group was set up in Autumn 1991 to formulate an overall assessment package and in particular the use of videotape consultations in summative assessment. They decided that the attributes of the ideal system should be:

- The trainer's assessment should carry weight
- There must be an objective external contribution
- Clinical competence must be directly assessed
- Performance throughout the year should count in the assessment
- A 100% pass rate should be possible
- Procedure must be feasible.

In terms of face validity it was considered that the ability of the doctor to carry out consultations successfully is a major determinant of overall competence. The group set out to define competence in broad but precise terms. The work was led by Dr Malcolm Campbell and reported in detail.

The working group decided to use four components in the assessment process:

• A multiple true-false paper

• Trainer's overall judgment

• A completed audit carried out by the trainee

• An assessment of the videotape consultations.

The group thought that each of the four components had specific features that would combine to produce a balanced overall assessment. Factual knowledge is obviously important in general practice. A properly constructed multiple choice paper is a reliable and feasible method of identifying factual knowledge. The aim was to use criterion referencing where possible and in the true-false multiple choice minimum levels of performance were decided by the group.

The trainer is uniquely placed to observe the trainee over the course of the year, particularly in the areas of attitudes and behaviour. It was acknowledged, however, that the trainer's judgment will be based, to some extent, on his or her previous experience of trainees and to that extent will contain elements of peer referencing. Performance review has long been recognised as a necessary component of the practice of medicine, and a completed audit will demonstrate that the trainee has absorbed the principles of audit and carried out the practice of performance review. The audit will be judged by using predefined criteria.

An audit project has been chosen because all general practitioners should be monitoring and improving the quality of care they provide. The ability to carry out an audit is therefore a skill of minimum competence for a GP registrar.

The major part of general practice takes place in the consultation with the individual patient. For any system of assessment to be credible it must cover this area. The use of videotaped consultations has potential advantages. It enables observation of real consultations in a relatively unobtrusive way. Tapes can be assessed by several assessors thereby measuring reliability and also calibrating the assessors. The group decided that the number of videotape assessors should be small to reduce variability but large enough to keep the workload to manageable proportions.

A registrar who is rated as satisfactory in all components would automatically receive a certificate of completion. A GP registrar who failed in any one area would enter a referral process. In this referral process the registrar's competence would be discussed by the regional adviser with the associate adviser and the trainer. A review of the registrar's portfolio would be undertaken by a further two assessors, at least one of whom would be from outside the region. When the system becomes national both final assessors will be from outside the region. If at the end of the process the trainee is deemed not to be competent the certificate of satisfactory completion would be refused and suitable additional training would be recommended.

The video is a powerful tool in assessing competence, and those who were royal college examiners thought that the ability to watch trainees consult went a long way towards the goal of assessing performance rather than competence. For each consultation a decision is made as to whether that consultation is an R+ which is a clear refer, R is a refer, P is a pass, and P+ is a clear pass. The assessor looks for the presence of minor errors or a major error. Criteria for listening are that the doctor identifies and illustrates reasons for attendance. A credible, acceptable plan should be negotiated. Action is also important with appropriate action taken to identify the patient's problem with reasonable investigation, referrals, and help sought when necessary, and with the patient's problem being managed appropriately. In terms of understanding, the trainee keeps a log to determine that he or she understands the process-outcome of the consultation. Actions are explained, obvious shortcomings identified, and relevant background mentioned.

Further work carried out has shown that a non-competent trainee would have a 95% probability of being identified by the process described. Each tape is reviewed individually by two assessors. The assessors had reached firm judgments by the time four consultations had been viewed, and the conclusion was that the use of videotaped consultations offers a feasible and reliable method of summative assessment.

The early multiple choice paper had an α coefficient of 0.76, and this rose to 0.8 after the removal of four items. The gold standard in any test sought by educationalists is

0.8. The paper concentrated on questions that were considered to be of relevance at the minimal acceptable competence – that is, they were questions to which acceptable trainees should know the answer.

The audit component was developed by Dr Murray Lough, and the criteria which are currently being used for marking the audits are:

- Reason for choice

- Criteria chosen

- Preparation and planning

- Interpretation of data

- Detailed proposals for change.

FORM FOR AUDIT

Question	Criterion	Criteria present
Why was the audit done?		
	Reason for choice	
	• Should be clearly defined and reflected in the title.	☐
	• Should include potential for change.	
How was the audit done?		
	Criteria chosen	
	• Should be relevant to the subject of the audit.	☐
	• Should be justified for example literature.	
	Preparation and planning	
	• Should show appropriate teamwork and methodology in carrying out audit.	☐
	• If standards are set they should be appropriate and justified.	
What was found?		
	Interpretation of data	
	• Should use relevant data to allow appropriate conclusions to be drawn.	☐
What next?		
	Detailed proposals for change	
	• Should show explicit details of proposed changes.	☐

A satisfactory GP registrar audit report must include all five criteria to pass
Fig. 7.1 Form for audit

By using the summative assessment process as developed in the west of Scotland about 5% of trainees were identified as not yet being competent to undertake independent practice. The trainer's opinion was the least discriminatory, and the following questions are now used:

- Clinical competence – Do you have any doubts about your trainee's clinical competence to perform unsupervised general practice? (yes/no)

- Professionalism – Does the trainee have an appropriate approach to the areas of confidentiality, continuing education, and relationships with colleagues, staff, and patients? (yes/no/doubtful)

- Reliability – Does the trainee behave in a responsible manner with regard to duties within the practice such as surgeries and home visits? (yes/no/doubtful)

- Personal organisation – Do you think the trainee will be able to cope with the organisational difficulties of general practice, particularly time management? (yes/no/doubtful)

- Other areas – Are there any other areas where you have doubts about the trainee's fitness for independent practice? (yes/no) If yes please specify.

If you think the trainee has difficulties in any of these areas please give details here.

United Kingdom summative assessment

The United Kingdom conference of regional advisers has now worked out a summative assessment programme for all regions for 1996. The factual knowledge and problem solving component is now being developed, and a question bank is now available and run on a national basis. The work on the submission of practical work is an audit that uses the system developed in the west of Scotland. The evaluation of clinical and consulting skills is using the system developed within the west of Scotland, and the trainer's overall opinion is a more detailed form which is currently being developed by the Oxford region.

Structured trainer's report

The trainer's report has been developed after a national survey of trainers' views. The standards were produced by a consensus group of experienced trainers. When the standards are reached the general practitioner registrar is considered to be ready for independent practice.

The report is divided into six sections:

- Patient care (itself divided into general clinical skills, patient management skills, and clinical judgment)

- Communication skills

- Personal and professional growth

- Organisational skills

- Professional values

- Specific clinical skills (this section includes a number of basic diagnostic and therapeutic skills).

Trainers are also given guidance as to the best method of assessment under three categories:

- Assessment by observation

- Assessment by discussion

- Assessment by specific methods.

All items will need to be completed satisfactorily for the report to be submitted, two months before the completion of training. Trainers have been instructed that whenever there is any doubt about whether or not the GP registrar has reached the necessary standard, repeat observation should be made. Clearly when a trainer is aware that a GP registrar is as yet unable to reach the required standard they will arrange for the appropriate training to occur and ask the advice of a course organiser, associate, or regional adviser.

What is the role of trainers in summative assessment and how are they being prepared?

All trainers will have been briefed within their regions regarding all components of summative assessment. The trainer's primary role is to ensure that the registrar is being given the best chance of passing. They will be highlighting any concerns as early as possible in the registrar year so that action

73

can be taken. The trainer will enlist the support of others if a registrar is not likely to pass all items. Registrars will then have the support of their trainer, course organiser, and associate or regional adviser in reaching the required standard.

MRCGP examination

The MRCGP examination is undergoing changes to meet the requirements of summative assessment. To date it has been a peer referenced examination with a built in pass rate of 75%. An appraisal of clinical and consulting skills will be added to the assessment of factual knowledge and problem solving within the examination. The college examiners will develop and evaluate a method for assessing clinical and consulting skills, and this will become part of the examination in the latter part of 1996.

As the royal college has not defined its consulting skills the pathway to certification now is as shown in figure 7.2.

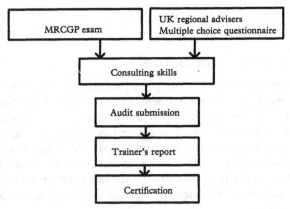

Figure 7.2

Summary

A description has been given of the development within the west of Scotland of a valid, reliable and feasible system of summative assessment for independent practice as a general practitioner. The development of summative assessment has been described over a 15 year period with the rapid recent changes. These could be modified before the final implementation date.

Further reading

General Medical Services Committee. *Your choices for the future. A survey of GP opinion.* London: General Medical Services Committee, 1992.

Royal College of General Practitioners. *Education and training for general practice. College policy statement.* London: Royal College of General Practitioners, 1994.

National Association of Health Authorities and Trusts. *Partners in learning, developing postgraduate training and continuing education for general practice.* London: NAHAT, 1994.

Campbell LM, Howie JGR, Murray TS. Summative assessment: a pilot project in the West of Scotland. *Br J Gen Pract* 1993; **43**: 430–4.

Campbell LM, Howie JGR, Murray TS. The use of videotaped consultations in summative assessment of trainees in General Practice. *Br J Gen Pract* 1995; **45**: 137–41.

Lough JRM, McKay J, Murray TS. Audit and summative assessment: 2 years pilot experience. *Medical Education* 1995; **29**: 101–3.

Lough JRM, McKay J, Murray TS. Audit and summative assessment: a criterion referenced marking schedule. *Br J Gen Pract* 1995; **45**: 607–9.

Campbell LM, Murray TS. Summative assessment in the west of Scotland: 3 year experience. *Br J Gen Pract* (in press).

Joint Committee on Postgraduate Training for General Practice. *Report of working party on assessment.* London: JCPTGP, 1993.

8 Examination for membership of the Royal College

The MRCGP examination has almost 2000 candidates a year. The exam became the only route to membership of the college in 1968, having been voluntary for a few years before. In the college publication which is a guide for candidates and teachers Pereira Gray lists five reasons why general practitioners should take the MRCGP examination.

Personal satisfaction – Passing the exam brings considerable personal and professional pride to young doctors, and they also receive the seal of approval from the royal college that they have reached a high standard. Their satisfaction is also considered important by all those who are concerned in their training process.

Career advancement – All those who aspire to leading positions within general practice need to have passed the examination.

Quality marker – The exam is currently peer referenced with a constant 75% passing. Success means that the examinee has reached a quality standard.

Financial advantage – The possession of membership may mean cheaper medical insurance with some of the professional indemnity services.

Supporting the discipline – Being a member of the college is part of the collective professional responsibility of general practitioners to support their royal college.

Who can sit?

Fully registered medical practitioners who have completed, or who will complete within 8 weeks of the date of the oral examination, three years' full time post registration experience may sit the exam. This must include either not less than two years in general practice or one year as a registrar and two years of full time medical experience, all within the United Kingdom and Eire or especially recognised by the college.

The training requirement is exactly that required for successful completion of vocational training. Details of the examination and an application form can be obtained from the membership department of the royal college, and applications normally have to be made at least 2 ½ months before the date of the examination. The dates are published frequently, and any candidate should check on those.

When the exam is applied for certificates of competence are required for cardiopulmonary resuscitation and child health surveillance. For cardiopulmonary resuscitation hospital specialists in accident and emergency or anaesthetics can provide a candidate with a certificate, or this can be also carried out by someone with specific skills. This could include general practitioners or training officers in the ambulance service. All candidates are required to produce evidence of their competence in the practical aspects of child health surveillance, and this certification can be carried out by principals in general practice who are carrying out this procedure on a regular basis and approved by their relevant family health services authority or health board to do so. Other doctors such as community paediatricians and clinical medical officers are also acceptable.

The examiners

MRCGP examiners are full time general practitioners who have an interest in education. They either offer themselves as examiners or are suggested by their colleagues. They must undertake specific training and must sit the exam and reach a level of achievement which is comparable with candidates reaching the oral stages of the examination. They then undergo regular training both during the examination by video, feedback, and observation. They also attend an annual examiner workshop.

The exam itself

The written components

There are three components in the written examination: the multiple choice question paper, the modified essay question paper, and the critical reading question paper. The examination is based on the job description of the general practitioner and the content of general practice as defined in *The Future General Practitioner – Learning and Teaching*. The examination is orientated towards practice in Britain within the NHS. The areas of knowledge assessed in the examination are as follows:

Clinical practice/health and disease – The candidate will be required to demonstrate a knowledge of the diagnosis, management, and, where appropriate, the prevention of diseases of importance in general practice.

- The range of the normal
- The patterns of illness
- The natural history of diseases
- Prevention
- Early diagnosis
- Diagnostic methods and techniques
- Management and treatment.

Clinical practice/human development – The candidate will be expected to possess a knowledge of human development and be able to demonstrate the value of this knowledge in the diagnosis and management of patients in general practice.

- Genetics
- Fetal development
- Physical development in childhood, maturity, and aging
- Intellectual development in childhood, maturity, and aging
- Emotional development in childhood, maturity, and aging
- The range of the normal.

Clinical practice/human behaviour – The candidate must demonstrate an understanding of human behaviour, particularly as it affects the presentation and management of disease.

- Behaviour presented to the general practitioner
- Behaviour and interpersonal relationships
- Behaviour of the family

- Behaviour in the doctor-patient relationship.

Medicine and society – The candidate must be familiar with the common sociological and epidemiological concepts and their relevance to medical care and demonstrate a knowledge of the organisation of medical and related services in the United Kingdom and abroad.

- Sociological aspects of health and illness
- The uses of epidemiology
- The organisation of medical care in the United Kingdom; comparisons with other countries
- The relation of medical services to other institutions in society
- Ethics
- Historical perspectives of general practice

The practice – The candidate must demonstrate a knowledge of practice organisation and administration and be able to discuss critically recent developments in the evolution of general practice.

- Practice management
- The team
- Financial matters
- Premises and equipment
- Medical records
- Medicolegal matters
- Research.

The examination is designed to assess, in various ways, the candidate's skills in:

- Interpersonal communication
- History taking
- Information gathering
- Selecting tests by using investigations and procedures
- Recording information
- Interpreting information
- Problem definition and hypothesis formation
- Early diagnosis
- Defining the range of intervention
- Selecting treatment
- Providing continuing care
- Interventive and preventive medicine in relation to the patient, the family, and the community

- Practice and personal organisation
- Teamwork, delegation, and relating to other colleagues
- Business matters
- Communications.

The candidate will be expected to demonstrate appropriate attitudes to patients, colleagues, and to the role of the general practitioner. The ability to develop and extend knowledge and skills through continuing education must be demonstrated.

This is an inclusive list reflecting the breadth of general practice, and specific preparatory books can be a great help.

The multiple choice question (MCQ paper)

The multiple choice question paper is designed to test the extent of the candidate's knowledge. This part of the examination is under continuous development to improve its reliability and relevance to contemporary medicine. A sound basis of knowledge and information about general practice is regarded by the examiners as an essential requirement for any good family doctor. Each question in the paper is intended to explore a topic in which an ordinary, well informed general practitioner could be expected to have a working knowledge. The paper is in two sections. The first section contains questions of the multiple true or false variety. These consist of a statement or stem followed by items, any or all of which may be true or false. The number of items per question will vary from three to six. There will be about 420 true or false items in all. The number of items in each subject area will be approximately:

- General medical problems (including locomotor) – 180
- External medicine (dermatology, ophthalmology, ear, nose, and throat – 60
- Women's health – 60
- Child health – 60
- Service management – 60.

Questions appear in random order in the paper.

The second section contains questions of the extended matching variety. These typically consist of a scenario which has to be matched to an answer from a list of options, but the candidate should read carefully the specific instruction for each question. For any one item he or she must choose one and only one of the options. There will usually be more options than items so not all of the options will be used. A given option may provide the answer to more than one item – for example, there might be two items which contain descriptions of patients and the most likely diagnosis could be the same in both instances. In this case the option would be used more than once. The candidate may think there are several possible answers to an item but he or she

---

Box 8.1 Example of extending matching question

Reduced vision in the eye

Options
a) Basilar migraine
b) Cerebral tumour
c) Cranial arteritis
d) Macular degeneration
e) Occlusion of the central retinal artery
f) Occlusion of the central retinal vein
g) Demyelinating optic neuritis
h) Retinal detachment
I) Tobacco optic neuropathy

Instruction: For each patient with reduced vision, select the most likely diagnosis. Each option can be used once, more than once, or not at all. Select only one option for each item.

Items:
1 A 75 year old man who is a heavy smoker, with blood pressure of 170/105 mm Hg complains of floaters in the right eye for many months and flashing lights in bright sunlight. He has now noticed a "curtain" across his vision in the right eye.
2 A 70 year old woman complains of shadows, which sometimes obscure her vision for a few minutes. She has felt unwell recently with loss of weight and face pain when chewing food.
3 A 45 year old woman, who is a heavy smoker, with blood pressure of 170/110 mm Hg, complains of impaired vision in the left eye. She has difficulty discriminating colours and has noticed that her eyes ache when looking to the side.

Answers
1 H
2 C
3 G

---

must choose the one most likely from the option list. Pictorial data, such as charts and photographs, may be included in the extended matching questions. There will be up to 90 extended matching items in all. These will cover a range of subject matters in general practice though not necessarily in the same proportions as the true or false items. The scoring of both parts is the same. Candidates are awarded one mark for each item answered correctly. Marks are not deducted for incorrect answers nor for failure to answer. The total score on the paper is the number of correct answers given. The candidate is therefore advised to attempt all items.

The MCQ is under constant development. Each question paper will contain a number of untested items which are included for trialing purposes. There may be different versions of the paper in which the tested items differ. These items will not be used in calculating the total score and up to 20% of the items may be of this type. They will appear in random order – for example, they will not necessarily be the last items on the paper.

The trialing of items in this way ensures that those items which are scored have been thoroughly tested and will produce a reliable result.

The extended matching questions test the candidates' ability to apply their knowledge to those situations which are likely to be found in practice and to apply probability in making diagnostic decisions.

Modified essay questions (MEQ paper)

The modified essay question paper examines the candidates' ability to integrate and apply theoretical knowledge and professional values within the setting of primary health care in the United Kingdom. It tests the candidates in:

- Skills and problem solving
- Prioritising and decision making in a wide range of clinical settings
- Insight into the psychological processes affecting the patient and the doctor and the relationship between them
- Recognition of the family, social, occupational, environmental, and cultural factors in the context of ill health
- Communication and consultation skills
- Understanding of the principles of preventive medicine and the promotion of good health

- Attitudes to patients, colleagues, and staff
- Appropriate use of resources including drugs, treatment facilities, referral agencies, other members of the health care team, ancillary staff, and complementary practitioners
- Familiarity with the general practitioner's role in practice organisation, administration, and management
- Appreciation of ethical principles on the general practitioner's terms of service
- Awareness of current or foreseeable trends and developments in primary care.

The MEQ paper consists of 12 questions to be answered in three hours. The paper includes a series of cameos such as might be encountered during a working day in practice with a question based on each. Candidates should base their time equally among all questions. As the answer paper is divided among examiners

---

Box 8.2 Example of MEQ with construct

A 35 year-old schoolteacher, Paul Wright, presents with a four day history of cough, wheeze, and copious green sputum. There is no significant history and on examination he has expiratory rhonchi but no signs of consolidation. Outline and explain your management.

Construct

1 *Further investigation considered* – Peak expiratory flow useful; radiography and sputum culture probably not much help

2 *Diagnostic possibilities* – Patient may have asthma or acute bronchitis, or both. Not possible at this stage to know which

3 *Treatment* – If peak expiratory flow is down, use of inhaled β adrenergic would be appropriate; if peak expiratory flow is down to < 60% oral steroids. Most general practitioners would consider prescribing an antibiotic as well, although doubtful if strictly necessary. Amoxycillin or erythromycin use should be considered

4 *Follow up* – Patient should be reviewed in one to two weeks, ideally with peak flow chart to see if it is asthma, for specific purposes of full diagnosis and decisions about further treatment

each question should be answered specifically with no reference to any other part of the answer.

The answer to each question is evaluated for its grasp of a number of independent constructs. Separate competencies which good practice requires are needed for a comprehensive response to the question. Examples of constructs include: sound clinical judgment, cost-effectiveness, insight, empathy and caritas, self awareness, and predictive ability. The good candidate reads each question carefully and answers it as asked; thinks in a wide ranging way but realistically about how a competent and sensitive general practitioner would deal with each scenario; avoids jargon, cliché, and overgeneralisation; and uses illustrative details, explanations, and relevant examples. The MEQ is a test of the candidate's practical approach to general practice problems, and as such candidates will gain more marks for their management of the problem than for their pure factual knowledge.

Critical reading question (CRQ paper)

The critical reading question paper is intended to assess the candidates in the following:

- Ability to evaluate published material relevant to general practice
- Ability to analyse and use data relevant to general practice
- Ability to base clinical and management decisions on published scientific evidence
- Familiarity with issues of importance in general practice and the ability to evaluate the different views and opinions published in the general practice literature
- Ability to apply clinical epidemiology to general practice.

The CRQ paper comprises 10 questions to be answered in three hours. Candidates should divide their time almost equally between all questions. The paper contains two sections. The first is entitled *reading on current practice* and is designed to test knowledge and interpretation of general practice literature. Most of the marks available will be awarded for demonstrating an understanding of the current views on a topic and the general evidence on which they are based. The candidate is expected to be familiar with items in the medical literature which have influenced current thinking on relevant issues in general practice. Candidates in their preparation should read reputable journals in a broadly based way. The advice is to study common clinical problems with general practice themes and search the literature for these rather than reading recent consecutive packages of journals. This preparation should take place throughout the training year, and references from reputable journals and books should be mentioned if they are relevant to the arguments being presented.

The second section is entitled *critical appraisal* and tests the candidate's ability to evaluate and interpret presented written material. This material may be in the form of published papers or extracts from papers, such as summaries or methods and results sections on their own. It may also include data relevant to general practice such as a protocol, a report, an audit, or a series of clinical results. The type of material presented in this section on the question asked is varied.

When the written papers are marked all those whose scores are more than 1 SD below the mean mark (around 85% of candidates) are invited for orals.

First oral

This is based on the practice experience questionnaire and is devoted to aspects of practice organisation and a discussion of the candidate's own patients. The candidate would be expected to defend the diagnosis and management of the situations described, and this oral examines clinical skills, as well as attitudes towards patients, colleagues, general practice, and the profession of medicine as a whole.

Second oral

In this examination the candidate is presented with various clinical problems and topics from general practice. Brief details of a patient may be provided with an outline of the presenting symptoms. Candidates will then be expected to describe their approach to the problem, seek further information from the examiners, outline the examination and investigations they would arrange, and demonstrate their ability to clarify the problem and reach a diagnosis. In this examination the candidate may be questioned on any topic.

There are seven areas of competence covered in the oral examinations.

- Problem definition
- Management
- Prevention
- Practice organisation
- Communication
- Professional values
- Personal and professional growth.

The examiners will try to cover as many of these as they can in the 30 minutes, and they will be looking for the attributes above. Candidates should have a range of reasonable alternative responses to a given situation. They should show an understanding of the actions they have taken or advised. The reasons for their actions should be well argued and supported by evidence where possible. They can be flexible in their attitudes, when appropriate, and their behaviour should be consistent with their expressed attitudes. At the end of the examination each examiner of the orals makes a judgment.

The five components each contribute one fifth of the total and any candidate who achieves an aggregate of 50% overall will pass. Although it is not intended to have a fixed proportion of successes, it is usual for about 75% of candidates to pass at each stage.

The future

From 1996–7 all candidates who are successful in the MRCGP will have had to have been successful in their summative assessment at the end of vocational training. The winter examination in 1996 will include a consultation skills model. Each candidate will submit a four hour video tape, which will be accompanied by a work book, and for each consultation the candidate will describe the presenting complaint, the relevant background information, outcomes of the consultation, and a comment about their performance in the consultation giving reasons as to why things went well or badly. The candidate will also describe any special features of the consultation. For each consultation they will also carry out a consultation map dealing with the specific tasks of clinical history, examination, patient's beliefs, effects of problem, continuing problems, health promotion, action taken, explanation, and management discussion. A method of marking has been devised consisting of certain performance criteria – that is, elements which were considered to be necessary for the performance to be judged as adequate. Some of these criteria will be deemed desirable with others essential. The level for pass or fail will be considerably above the minimal competence expected in summative assessment.

The MRCGP is the quality marker of achievement at the end of vocational training. Preparation for the examination should be throughout the trainee year with a particular effort being made in the few months before.

Further reading

Moore R. *The MRCGP examination.* London: Royal College of General Practitioners, 1994.

Elliott P. *MRCGP MCQ practice papers.* Knutsford: PASTEST, 1993.

Saunders J. *MRCGP practice examinations.* 2nd ed. Knutsford: PASTEST, 1992.

Royal College of General Practitioners. *Examination for membership of the Royal College of General Practitioners (MRCGP).* London: RCGP, 1990. (Occasional Paper No 46.)

Murray TS. *Modified essay questions for the MRCGP examination.* 2nd ed. Oxford: Blackwell, 1995.

Jones R, Kinmouth A. *Critical reading for primary care.* Oxford: Oxford University Press, 1995.

Ridsdale L. *Evidence based general practice. A critical reader.* London: Saunders, 1995.

9 Continuing medical education, postgraduate education allowance, and professional development

It is important to define adult and professional learning. Adult learning is purposeful, voluntary, and initiated by adults themselves. A great deal of how this is arranged will be based on their previous experience, their own learning agenda, and their self esteem.

There are three widely accepted characteristics of a profession which are important in this context. Firstly, competence – professions claim the right of control over entry to their own membership and with this goes the obligation to be accountable for the competence of that membership. Secondly, judgment – within professions members' decisions depend on expert judgments of individual practitioners and they cannot be made on the basis of standardised rules, thus learning to be a professional includes the development of the powers of judgment. In terms of adult learning professional learners need to discover how to exercise expert professional judgment for themselves. Thirdly, the nature of the work – that is, professional learning which depends on two main things, knowledge and skill. The skill needed for a profession is based on a well established body of theoretical knowledge which is then applied to specific problems.

Box 9.1 Characteristics of a profession

- Competence
- Judgment
- Professional learning

In an address on the importance of postgraduate study Osler commented, "If the licence to practice meant the completion of his education, how sad it would be for the practitioner, how distressing to his patients! More clearly than any other the physician should illustrate the truth of Plato's saying that education is a lifelong process. The training of the medical school gives a man his direction, points him in the way and furnishes a chart fairly incomplete for the voyage, but nothing more".

The seeds of the present day structure were sown in 1961 at a memorable conference on postgraduate medical education held at Christchurch, Oxford. The Christchurch conference was notable because of the catalytic effect it had on the development of postgraduate medicine within regions and districts of the NHS and in particular the growth of what came to be described as a postgraduate medical centre movement.

Two surveys on general practitioners' views on continuing medical education were carried out in 1974. In the north east of Scotland 217 general practitioners responded to a questionnaire in which they expressed a preference for single week courses covering several subjects and including a mixture of lectures, case presentations, and group discussions. Only 18% thought that lunch time meetings were acceptable as a source of regular education. The respondents rated contact with their partners and hospital colleagues as the most important source of education, and it was thought that this link had to be the growth point for postgraduate education within an integrated health service.

In England and Wales a questionnaire was sent to a randomly selected sample of 1904 general practitioners. There were 1067 respondents representing 5.3% of all practitioners in England and Wales. Respondents preferred long intensive courses and thought the dissemination of information about national courses was defective. A third of those required a locum in order to attend a course but had difficulty in obtaining one. The survey also showed that local educational activity was enhanced by the presence of a postgraduate medical centre.

An extensive survey was carried out in the northern region in 1979 with a precoded questionnaire being sent to a 50% random sample of the 1328 general practitioner principals in that region. Of the 664 questionnaires sent, 499 were returned, giving a response rate of 75.2%. The respondents' perceptions of postgraduate education were sought and their behaviour measured by the number of sessions they had attended during the previous year at both their usual and other postgraduate centres. Only 4% had not attended any postgraduate events during the previous year, but the remaining respondents had attended eight sessions on average, six of which were at their usual centres. Those attending more than the average number of sessions tended to have registered between 1950 and 1969, work in larger practices, hold additional appointments, or be trainers or college tutors.

A survey in 1980 suggested that continuing education for general practice was not given the attention that it deserves. At this time looking at the research into continuing medical education the authors noted that there was no established research tradition of general practitioners' continuing education as the volume of published research on the subject had been small, and in the early 1980s there were no signs of it increasing quickly.

The Leeuwenhorst European working party on continuing education for general practitioners noted that the aims of continuing education were concerned with the maintenance, development, and improvement of the care which doctors provide for people through their professional life and which starts for general practitioners when they assume professional responsibility. This would still be true today. The 1980 working party suggested that its purpose should be:

- To review knowledge, skills, and attitudes already acquired in undergraduate and vocational training, eliminating those which are obsolete while retaining those which are still valuable.
- To help doctors to discover their deficiencies and to deal with

the difficulties which they already recognise in their own work by sharing experiences with their colleagues both medical and non-medical

- To help doctors to recognise and apply new evidence and ideas by using the experience of general practice as a basis for their evaluation and application; by giving as well as receiving training in this way they will be enabled to develop new competencies and learn new roles effectively
- To help doctors' capacity to think creatively and to appraise their own work critically by means of education and research activities.

Box 9.2 Retaining appropriate knowledge, skills and attitudes

- Discover deficiencies and share experiences with colleagues
- Recognise and apply new evidence using general practice experience as a vehicle
- Develop new competencies and learn new roles
- Think creatively and appraise own work

Studies in the early 80s suggested that only a small number of general practitioners had poor motivation towards their own continuing education, but 82% had encountered difficulties as a result of lack of time, practice commitments, and the need to preserve family life. Other problems which were mentioned were poor communications about courses, inconvenient timing, distance from practice, locum difficulties, and lack of motivation. In 1984 a random one in five survey of Scottish general practitioners produced an 80% response. Of the preferred learning methods, reading at home was rated the most highly by 73% of the doctors. In relation to the educational content recent medical advances with diagnosis and treatment of disease were supported by 82% of the respondents while clinical developments in general practice were favoured by 62%.

The most common adverse comment related to provisions for continuing education with regard to the special difficulties encountered by isolated doctors and their inability to find adequate time for continuing education due to overwork. Further work tended to reinforce the work already quoted.

Horder, quoting from a literature review, thought that valid and convincing evidence of the efficacy of continuing education was not plentiful. There was a widespread belief in education as a method influencing general practitioners, but gains in knowledge and skill with resultant changes in behaviour seemed harder to achieve with general practitioners than with undergraduates. He noted that the difficulties increased with the age of the practitioner and were likely to accelerate from the age of 40. Deficiencies identified in this group were more likely to be in performance than in knowledge.

A *BMJ* editorial in 1987 stated that continuing medical education must not be an optional extra and that the standard of care offered by a doctor was related less to his or her knowledge than to factors affecting its application, and the most important of these was motivation. Doctors need to know what they are trying to do and how well they are doing it to maintain their enthusiasm otherwise they develop rituals and their performance declines. A *Lancet* editorial at the same time noted a growing awareness that traditional continuing education was seldom effective in changing doctors' attitudes and their adaptability. Although general practitioners had been especially concerned about the need for a new approach to continuing education, progress was painfully slow and there had been no serious attempt to devise clear strategies.

A royal college occasional paper on continuing education in 1988 thought that the findings for continuing education were

---

Box 9.3 Wider role of continuing medical education

- Maintaining interests
- Encouraging high professional standards
- Keeping up to date
- Motivating
- Providing reassurance
- Comparison with others
- Boosting confidence

---

quite profound insofar as they pointed to the differing needs of different groups of doctors and suggested opportunities for continuing education courses to play a wider part than merely imparting information. These included maintaining interest, encouraging high professional standards and the ethos of being up to date, stimulating and motivating, providing reassurance, enabling contact, comparison with other doctors, and enhancing group identity and confidence.

A study in Wales in 1989 that carried out in depth interviews with doctors found that general practitioners considered the most beneficial educational activities occurred within the practice, the most valued being contact with partners. They also asked for increased contact with hospital doctors. Further work at this time pointed out that there was no mention of assessing the value of courses. The regional advisers, on looking at their future strategy in 1989, looked at the guiding educational principles, the educational needs of general practitioners, the provisions required, the management processes, and the infrastructure. They also considered some of the likely political changes. Parry in 1990 in an article on effective continuing medical education thought that three issues were relatively new: firstly, the search for good standards in general practice; secondly, renewed interest in the need to understand the stress under which general practitioners work; and, finally, many younger general practitioners were becoming interested in the idea of a career in general practice. A study carried out after this time suggested that particular priority should be given to further training in new clinical treatments, staff development, computerisation, and clinical audit.

The 1990 contract, general practice in the NHS, prescribed that the existing training allowances would be replaced by a new postgraduate education allowance designed to encourage continuing medical education throughout a general practitioner's time in active practice. All costs, including tuition fees, would be reimbursed through fees and allowances but on an average basis. The document also noted that seniority payments would be retained but would be reduced by the value of the new postgraduate education allowance to which all general practitioners would be entitled provided they met the necessary training requirements, which entailed a balanced programme of continuing education. To claim the allowance general practitioners would have to submit evidence to their employing authority that they had attended an average of five days training a year over the previous five years. Although the general practitioner could vary the amount of time spent on courses from year to year, he or she would be expected to achieve a reasonable balance between the years. The government expected that this new allowance would stimulate interest among educational organisations and lead to the availability of an increased variety of courses.

Box 9.4 Postgraduate education allowance

- Average of five days annually over a five year period
- Balanced approach

Categories:
- Health promotion
- Disease management
- Service management

To ensure that general practitioners would be able to keep up to date and extend their range of knowledge and skill in general practice activities, courses would be divided into three broad categories: health promotion and prevention of illness, disease management, and service management. To claim the allowance general practitioners would have to attend at least two courses under each of the three headings over the five years preceding the claim.

When the new contract was introduced the allowance was set at £1995, and from that the general practitioners had to pay the expenses element of their educational activities. The only aspect of education which continued to be centrally funded was vocational training for general practice which continued to be supported by section 63.

It was thought that these changes would create a competitive environment for continuing education in which doctors and their staff would choose courses as purchasers would choose any commodity on the basis of usefulness, attraction, cost-effectiveness, etc. Many providers of education emerged, and the traditional sources – for example postgraduate centres and universities – came under increasing competitive and economic pressures.

The regional advisers in their strategic document noted that one of the government's aims was to guarantee the quality of courses and activities by ensuring that they were accredited as educationally valuable and recommended to general practitioners by the regional adviser in general practice. They noted that the impact of the scheme on an individual general practitioner was that the underlying concept was one of transferring educational choice and responsibility in continuing medical education to the individual general practitioner. In theory they thought doctors would use their allowance to seek out and pay for those courses they considered best suited to their needs. Others were concerned that there may be an attempt to take the cheapest option with a return to traditional lectures.

Papers during the subsequent years noted the increase in activity, although there was some questioning of the appropriateness of some. The occasional paper on portfolio based learning expressed disappointment that the new arrangements did little or nothing to foster continuing medical education on accepted principles of adult learning. An educational scheme was set up in the west of Scotland to cope with the new arrangements. This allowed examination of the factors influencing the uptake of continuing medical education among general practitioners and also allowed their educational achievements and characteristics to be studied over a three year period.

Previous literature had stated concern about the uptake of continuing education among general practitioners, and in the first year of this new allowance almost 95% of general practitioners attended sufficient meetings to claim the allowance. Initially meetings which were contract based or related were the most popular with service management, and health promotion was more popular than disease management. With regard to timing of the meetings, evenings were preferred when a large range of options was given.

One hundred and two doctors (5.7%) did not claim their first allowance. These doctors were more likely to work in urban areas, be single handed, and have qualified more than 30 years ago. One hundred and seventy one (9.5%) were high attenders and were more likely to work in urban areas, be women, be members of the royal college, and work in a training practice. They were between 10 and 30 years from qualification and worked in larger group practices. There was considerable variation in the educational credits obtained by general practitioners with 4.2% completing more than double the requirement.

Within the region doctors attended in excess of what was required by the new regulations and met the category provisions which were defined in the statement of fees and allowances. A regional package with an annual charge was a viable and popular option to meet the requirements of the postgraduate education allowance.

Despite the changes in the delivery of continuing medical education doctors continued to attend courses outside their own region. The centrally organised educational scheme for the region was more likely to give a balanced spread and to meet the educational requirements of the 1990 contract. This was true for all three categories but was particularly true for health promotion and service management. Over the period of the study the following factors had a small but significant bearing on attendance: location of practice, whether working full time or part time or in a training practice, marital status, and being a member of the royal college. This information is important to primary care departments and others concerned in the delivery of health care and also to organisers of educational meetings.

The uptake of continuing medical education by general practitioners was greatly affected by the educational changes in the 1990 contract. These changes stimulated a considerable interest in education and resulted in an increased variety of courses.

The crux of continuing education is whether attending meetings affects the way a doctor works and delivers health care. Do doctors who attend more meetings bring greater benefits to their patients? Recent work has shown that attending meetings does increase knowledge in most cases and that this is truer for disease management than the other two categories. The acquisition of knowledge, however, and the level of change which this brings within the practice is disappointingly low. Overall the level of change which is achieved is small and seems to have little effect on the quality of care. As a result of this work the recommendation was that each doctor should develop a personal education plan, and this seems particularly true for single handed doctors in small practices, doctors in rural situations, doctors who are not in a training environment, and doctors who are not members of the royal college. These groupings seem the area of greatest need and with limited resources available are those with the greatest need for guidance. Gray, in 1986, examining what techniques are effective in continuing education, suggested that effective education should be based on the following principles:

- The education should be based on the doctor's own work as well as on research findings
- The doctor should be helped to assess his or her work and compare it with that of others
- The whole team should be involved where teamwork is necessary for good quality care
- Continuing education programmes should be developed in collaboration with doctors rather than being imposed on them
- The views of patients should be incorporated in continuing education
- Continuing education should help the physician not only to acquire new knowledge and skills but also to change the way he or she works
- Continuing education must be based on the assumption that doctors are busy and that nearly all would like to improve the quality of care they provide
- Doctors should be involved in the development of their continuing education and continuing education should be enjoyable.

Box 9.5 Effective education

- Based on doctor's own work
- Should compare work with that of others
- Whole team should be involved
- Should be involved in planning
- Patient's view is important
- Should affect health care
- Requires personal involvement

In their strategy document the regional advisers thought that the most fundamental change would be in an increased emphasis on a more personal practice based and targeted approach to continuing training and education. Their report considered that educational relevance, the effective approaches to learning, and the outcome of performance reviews both voluntary and statutory should underpin the process of planning, provision, and quality assurance in continuing education in general practice.

Pendleton in his 1995 William Pickles lecture illustrated the differences between academic and professional approaches to continuing medical education (table 9.1).

Table 9.1 Differences between academic and professional approaches to continuing medical education

Variable	Academic	Professional
Major aim	Insight and knowledge	Action to solve a problem
Urgency	Low	High
Cost-benefit analysis	Irrelevant	Crucial
Principal quality criterion	Elegance	Practicality
Usual source of insight	Own research, others' experience	Others' research, own experience
Level of complexity	High	Low
Means of persuasion	Theory backed by data	Data backed by argument
Preferred medium of presentation	Written	Face to face
Personality type most valued	Introvert	Extrovert
Method for dealing with uncertainty	Statistical	Personal

He also thought that regular strategic planning was crucial for professional development, and his plan for this is shown in figure 9.1.

The techniques for practice development were strategic planning workshops, team building with the techniques for individual development, peer review, focused audit, action plan, video based feedback on consultations and joint working.

This does illustrate the major problem at present with continuing education – that is, it does not deal with the learning needs of the participants. Despite many reports little has changed. An effective strategy for continuing medical education and

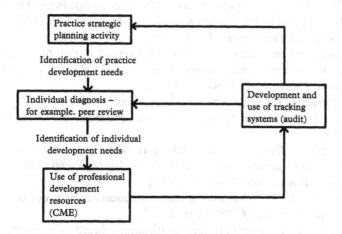

Figure 9.1 Strategic planning for professional development in general practice

continuing professional development is a high priority for the planners of these areas. The postgraduate education allowance, however, as currently constituted is not fulfilling this need.

Further reading

Pendleton D. Professional development in general practice, problems, puzzles and paradigms. *Br J Gen Pract* 1995; **45**: 377–81.

Osler W. The importance of postgraduate study. *Lancet* 1990; **ii**: 73–5.

Anon. 1962. Postgraduate medical education. Conference convened by the Nuffield Provincial Hospitals Trust. *Lancet* 1962; **i**: 367–8.

Durno D, Gill GM. Survey of general practitioners' views on postgraduate education in north east Scotland. *Journal of the Royal College of General Practitioners* 1974; **24**: 648–54.

Aitcheson HWK. Continuing education in general practice in England and Wales. *Journal of the Royal College of General Practitioners* 1974; **24**: 643–7.

Reedy BLEC, Gregson BA, Williams M. *General practitioners*

and *postgraduate education in the northern region*. London: Royal College of General Practitioners, 1979. (Occasional Paper No 9.)

Wood J, Bryne PS. *Section 63 activities*. London: Royal College of General Practitioners, 1980. (Occasional Paper No 11.)

Leeuwenhorst European Working Party. Continuing education and general practitioners. *Journal of the Royal College of General Practitioners* 1980; **30**: 570–4.

Donald AG. Continuing learning in practice project (CLIPP). *Journal of the Royal College of General Practitioners*. 1984; **34**: 242–5.

Horder J, Bosanquet N, Stocking B. Ways of influencing the behaviour of general practitioners. *Journal of the Royal College of General Practitioners* 1986; **36**: 517–21.

Schofield TPC. Continuing medical education must not be an optional extra. *BMJ* 1987; **294**: 526–7.

Editorial. Postgraduate and continuing education in need of orchestration. *Lancet* 1987; **ii**: 898–9.

Branthwaite A, Ross A, Henshaw A, Davie C. *Continuing education for general practitioners*. London: Royal College of General Practitioners, 1988. (Occasional Paper No 38.)

Owen PA, Allery LA, Harding KG, Hayes TM. General practitioners' continuing medical education within and outside their practice. *BMJ* 1989; **299**: 238–40.

England and Wales Working Party of Regional and Associate Regional Advisers in General Practice. *Future strategies for continuing medical education in general practice*. 1989

Parry KM. Effective continuing medical education. *Medical Education* 1990; **24**: 546–50.

RCGP Working Group on Higher Professional Education. *Portfolio based learning in general practice*. London: Royal College of General Practitioners, 1993. (Occasional Paper No 63.)

Health Departments of Great Britain. *General practice in the National Health Service – the 1990 contract*. London: HMSO, 1989.

Murray TS, Dyker GS, Campbell LM. Characteristics of general practitioners who did not claim the first postgraduate education allowance. *BMJ* 1991; **302**: 1377.

Murray TS, Dyker GS, Campbell LM. A regional programme in the west of Scotland to meet the demands of the postgraduate education allowance. *Postgraduate Education for General Practice* 1992; **3**: 62–4.

Murray TS, Dyker GS, Campbell LM. Characteristics of

general practitioners who are high attenders at educational meetings. *Br J Gen Pract* 1992; **42**: 157–9.

Murray TS, Dyker GS, Campbell LM. Postgraduate education allowance: general practitioners' attendance at courses outwith their region. *Br J Gen Pract* 1992; **42**: 194–6.

Murray TS, Dyker GS, Campbell LM. Continuing medical education and the education allowance: variations in credits obtained by general practitioners. *Medical Education* 1992; **26**: 248–350.

Murray TS, Dyker GS, Campbell LM. Postgraduate education allowance, a regional analysis of the first year. *Health Bulletin* 1992; **50(5)**: 348–50.

Murray TS, Dyker GS, Campbell LM. Postgraduate education allowance: educational attainment of subscribers and non-subscribers to a centrally organised educational scheme. *Br J Gen Pract* 1993; **43**: 19–21.

Murray TS, Dyker GS, Kelly MH, *et al.* Demographic characteristics of general practitioners attending educational meetings. *Br J Gen Pract* 1993; **43**: 467–9.

Kelly MH. *Evaluation of continuing medical education for general practitioners in the west of Scotland.* Glasgow: University of Glasgow, 1993. (PhD thesis).

10 Reaccreditation or recertification

In chapter 9 continuing medical education (CME) has been discussed, in particular those aspects relevant to general practice. To a professional person it is self evident that education is a lifelong commitment and that there is a continuing duty to keep up to date with modern medical developments. This commitment on the part of doctors is equally important to their patients who, in this consumerist era, are rightly ever more demanding of standards of clinical care.

This professional responsibility has been restated explicitly by

---

Box 10.1 Extract from *The Duties of a Doctor*, (GMC, 1995)

"You must maintain the standard of your performance by keeping your knowledge and skills up to date throughout your working life. In particular, you should take part regularly in educational activities which relate to your branch of medicine.

You must work with colleagues to monitor and improve the quality of health care. In particular you should take part in regular and systematic clinical audit.

Some parts of medical practice are governed by law. You must observe and keep up to date with the laws which affect your practice."

---

the GMC in its recent publication *The Duties of a Doctor* (box 10.1).

This obvious relation between professionals' duty towards education and high standards demanded by the public has been consummated in a marriage between them represented by the developing and important concept of reaccreditation.

There is a current debate whether the term reaccreditation or the term recertification is more appropriate. The GMSC prefers the former and the royal college the latter. For the purposes of this chapter the term reaccreditation will be used, but the process described by each body is almost exactly the same. The elements of reaccreditation are described in box 10.2.

Box 10.2 Elements of reaccreditation

Reaccreditation:
- Is a *professional* activity
- Has implications for *public accountability* and for *quality assurance*
- Renews and updates medical knowledge throughout professional life
- Identifies those whose standards are below an acceptable minimum and offers remedial educational activity

---

Reaccreditation as a professional activity

During the early years of the 1990s both the GMSC and the royal college recognised that the profession should be moving towards a system of structured education for the established practitioner and for some form of quality assurance within general practice. Because of public criticism of the variable quality within the discipline this could be seen as a defensive move; most general practitioners, however, have realised that change within medical practice has accelerated in recent years and that continuing medical education has never been more important for that reason alone.

Reaccreditation is only an echo of accreditation, which has also recently taken root with the development of summative assessment at the end point of vocational training (this is described further in chapter 7). General practice is not the only discipline that has started down this route, the Royal College of Obstetricians and Gynaecologists, the Royal College of Physicians of Edinburgh, and others have pioneered the use of continuing medical education as a method of reaccreditation, and it would seem likely that all doctors who enjoy the privilege of practising in an unsupervised environment, be they termed specialist, consultant, or general practitioner principal, will soon have to subscribe to such a system.

In the United States and Canada reaccreditation has been established over a long period, but the method used across the Atlantic has tended more towards the retrospective examination of medical records (chart review) and on review of clinical outcomes. In Canada, however, there have been more recent moves to incorporate a programme of postgraduate education as an integral part of the reaccreditation process.

The United Kingdom, on the other hand, has always tended towards the view that structured education is a more appropriate avenue of approach. For the vast majority of professionals in the United Kingdom, of course, reaccreditation is only a method of formalising the normal process of continuing medical education that they have previously voluntarily undertaken, and it will not come as a major professional hurdle – merely a trip wire for the incompetent. The GMC also proposes a system of professional review and remedial training for those whose standards have fallen to unacceptable levels, and its performance procedures are described later in this chapter.

Reaccreditation as a protection for the public

While doctors have willingly grasped the concept of adequate performance as a professional duty, reaccreditation does have implications for quality assurance for the patients they serve.

It is only since 1953 that newly graduated doctors with a basic medical degree have had to undertake additional preregistration training before "putting up their plate" as a general practitioner. In 1971 structured vocational training was introduced, and 1996–7 should see the universal application of summative assessment of that training. There is still, however, a great variation in the standard of general medical practice in the United Kingdom, and reaccreditation is merely an extension of the legitimate desire of a self regulating profession to ensure that its members are practising to acceptable standards.

It is axiomatic that minimum professional standards cannot be practised without the possession of a minimum amount of knowledge or skill, and continuing medical education is necessary both for their retention and for the acquisition of newer elements that are constantly thrown up by medical research and developments in practice. Attitudes in medical practice are perhaps less amenable to education and training, but deficiencies in this area should be dealt with by the GMC.

As described above, members of the general public also have a legitimate interest in reaccreditation and are major "stakeholders", therefore resources for its introduction should rightly attract public funds. The introduction of reaccreditation promises to require increased resources in terms of protected time for doctors to undertake the necessary education, in terms of the academic personnel required for a mentor based approach, and in terms of monitoring of the process.

Reaccreditation and medical knowledge

Intrinsic to the idea of continuing medical education is the recognition that new methods of medical education need to be used that concentrate on the adult learner (see chapter 9).

As with other adults, doctors develop different learning styles and, as they grow professionally, have differing learning needs. This implies that in contrast with undergraduate, basic professional, or even higher specialist training and education, established doctors require an approach that is individually tailored – that is, a personal education plan.

The personal education plan is one that will assess both the strengths and weaknesses in an individual and concentrate time and effort in making good the deficiencies, rather than subjecting all to the same curriculum. Such an approach suggests the use of an educational mentor who would not act as a teacher but who would tend to encourage reflection within each doctor as to where gaps in knowledge and skill lie and how best to seek to fill them. This is the basis of the concept promoted by the royal college of portfolio based learning.

In portfolio based learning, an assessment of individual learning needs is compiled, followed by a strategy for appropriate learning. This will depend on the individual's learning style. Learning styles have been identified recently by

Box 10.3 Learning styles (*Honey and Mumford* 1993)

Activists:

- Enjoy new experiences, problems or opportunities from which to learn
- Can engross themselves in short activities such as games, teamwork based tasks or role-playing exercises
- Enjoy excitement, drama, or crisis and can chop and change with diverse activities
- Can adopt a high visibility, can chair meetings, lead discussions, or give presentations
- Prefer to generate ideas without constraints of policy, structure, or feasibility
- Can cope with being "thrown in at the deep end"
- Enjoy involvement with other people and working as a team

Reflectors:

- Prefer to watch, think, and chew over activities
- Can stand back from events and listen and observe – "taking a back seat"
- Prefer to think before acting and to have time to assimilate and prepare
- Are able to carry out research; to investigate and assemble information and to probe to get to the bottom of things
- Prefer to review what has happened as a learning process
- React well to requests for carefully considered analyses and reports
- Prefer to react with other people within a structured learning environment
- Prefer to reach a decision in their own time without pressure and tight deadlines

Theorists:

- Prefer learning as part of a system, model, concept, or theory
- Prefer time to explore methodically the associations and inter-relationships between ideas, events, and situations
- Like the opportunity to question and probe basic methodologies
- Enjoy being intellectually stretched by analysing complex situations
- Prefer learning in a structured situation with a clear purpose
- Prefer to listen or read about ideas and concepts that have a logical basis
- Have the ability to analyse and then generalise the reasons for success or failure
- Enjoy being offered interesting ideas and concepts even though they are not immediately relevant
- Enjoy participation in complex situations

Pragmatists:

- Prefer there to be an obvious link between the subject matter and the problem
- Prefer to be shown techniques for doing things with obvious practical advantages
- Enjoy trying out and practising techniques with coaching from a credible expert
- Prefer a model they can emulate – for example a respected senior
- Prefer to be given techniques currently applicable to their own job
- Prefer to have immediate opportunities to implement what they have learned
- Prefer high "face validity" – that is good stimulation or "real" problems
- Prefer to concentrate on practical issues

two workers in the educational field and are described in box 10.3.

In 1993 the royal college published an occasional paper on this approach to learning and its application to general practice. The definition of the process and the steps involved are reproduced in box 10.4.

Box 10.4 Portfolio based learning (RCGP)

Portfolio based learning recognises:

- The value and significance of past learning and experience for the individual
- The ability of adults to act and learn autonomously
- The centrality of reflection in the learning process
- The need for meaningful links to be made between experiences, learning opportunities, and role requirements

The steps in the process of portfolio based learning are:

- Identification of experiences which the learner defines as significant – namely, important sources of learning
- Identification of what learning arose from these experiences and how that learning can be demonstrated in practice
- Identification of further learning needs, and ways in which these can be met

---

Reaccreditation and minimum standards

The prime purpose of reaccreditation is to assure professionals that their standards are at least at a level of minimum competence for independent practice and to give them the opportunity to improve even further – reinforcing the idea that even full and distinguished membership of a profession implies a lifelong status as a student. If it is universally applied, however, the process will also identify that small number within any profession whose standards have slipped sufficiently to call into question their continuing in practice.

Reaccreditation has the great advantage of detecting deteriorating trends in performance and of facilitating remedial action before a knowledge base declines to an irretrievable level, or even more importantly to a level where the professional becomes a danger to the public.

The new GMC performance procedures are described at the end of this chapter, but before the GMC becomes involved there is much that can be done informally through educational measures.

There is much work in the literature that suggests that educational opportunities are more often taken up voluntarily by those least in need of them, and the assessment of learning needs by reaccreditation promises a method of identifying those who are most in need of remedial education.

Models for reaccreditation

In recent years both the "service" and "academic" wings of general practice have examined the issue. In 1994 the annual conference of local medical committees, the policy making body for the GMSC, set out proposals. In 1993 a working party of the royal college's Scottish council made similar recommendations. These policies are listed in box 10.5.

Both the GMSC and the royal college have followed these policies on reaccreditation to ensure that all general practitioners are performing to a minimum standard, and the models proposed are described in box 10.6.

The GMSC plan is currently more developed in detail, but the two main bodies representing the interests of general practice have produced remarkably similar schemes. They are both based on voluntary participation initially, but with the eventual aim of universal application. Both bodies believe that the process should concentrate on the production of a minimum but ever rising standard of practice and on the remedial education of those falling below the minimum standard. Both schemes are predicated on the belief that the current arrangements for the postgraduate education allowance are ill targeted and that in future education for general practitioners should be based on individual needs. The royal college uses the term recertification but, in essence, it describes the same scheme as the GMSC. The GMSC has considered practice reaccreditation but for the time being has rejected it; the royal college's scheme encourages both individuals and practices to be involved. It must be hoped that the promotion of general practice to the centre of the NHS as proposed by the government's 1990 reforms will produce the

Box 10.5 Policy on reaccreditation/recertification	
GMSC policy	**RCGP policy**
Reaccreditation of individual general practitioners should:	Basic principles and aims:
• Be compulsory • Be personal • Identify any remedial action required • Be strictly confidential • Be simple to administer • Receive protected time • Probably be undertaken every five years • Be defined to the profession's satisfaction • Be professionally led with local medical committees having a specific input • Allow for the problems of inner city general practitioners • Be introduced after detailed agreement with the health departments • Be funded by new money outside the current pool	• To improve the basic knowledge, experience, and skills of general practitioners • To maintain a regular and organised system of renewing such knowledge and acquiring new skills and knowledge • To give individual general practitioners information on areas of competence and deficiency to plan future education • To promote the continual application of critical thought to everyday general practice • To maintain control of accreditation and postgraduate education within the profession • To influence postgraduate education to move towards areas of direct relevance and practicality to general practice

considerable financial and educational resources that these ambitious changes would require.

The GMC's performance procedures

The GMC has been cited earlier (box 10.1) with regard to the professional duty of doctors to keep their medical knowledge up to date. It has, of course, other functions relating to doctors' professional discipline and to the proper protection of the public from those who are, or have become, incompetent. Currently, the GMC has two "fitness to practise" procedures that apply to all

Box 10.6 The two models for reaccreditation/ recertification

GMSC model	RCGP model
• Five year rolling cycle	• Five year rolling cycle
• Professional mentor	• Examination based individual needs assessment
• Annual educational plan	
• "Compulsory", "negotiated", and "free" courses	• Individual and practice recertification
• Abolition of postgraduate education allowance, compulsory participation	• Practice questionnaire for practice assessment
• Extended practice visit if education in doubt	• Practice visit on "trainer approval" model
• Resources for protected educational time	• Postgraduate education allowance attendance revamped to satisfy individual need
• Resources for regional adviser infrastructure	• Standard setting by consensus, but rising standards
• National standards set by national body	• Failure of recertification leads to remedial action
• Failure of reaccreditation leads to remedial action	

doctors. The original, quasijudicial disciplinary procedure which was introduced by the Medical Act of 1858 (Professional Conduct) was supplemented in 1980 by the more humane approach to sick doctors enshrined in its health procedures.

In recent years, however, there has been much criticism of the GMC. Because a "conviction" under professional conduct procedures can lead to the loss of a doctor's livelihood the standard of proof required is necessarily high. Previously, the GMC was prevented from considering a pattern of many, less serious lapses in a doctor's conduct which often led to great public concern.

Under the new performance procedures, which are the subject of legislation that received Royal Assent in November 1995, such a pattern of poor professional behaviour will soon be able to be considered by a new "fitness to practise" committee which by mid-1997 will have the power to subject a doctor to assessment of performance and to recommend remedial education or training.

This can be seen as the final stage of reaccreditation and is where the poor performance of "failures" of the GMSC/royal college systems will be considered if earlier remedial action has failed. The difference between the GMC and the GMSC/royal college systems lies in the emphasis accorded to the twin aims of examining doctors' performance. The prime concern of the GMC will be the protection of the public, with the interests of the doctor being secondary; the GMSC/royal college scheme will concentrate on the needs of the doctor but will always have to consider danger to the public.

Given the absolute duty of a doctor always to consider the needs of patients, the end stage of any professional reaccreditation process which fails to secure an improvement in deficient performance will always have to be referral of the case for more formal GMC consideration.

Further reading

Burrows P. *Canada 1994: report on a three month sabbatical visit to McMaster University, Hamilton, Ontario.* Personal communication, 1994.

General Medical Council. *The duties of a doctor.* London: GMC, 1995.

General Medical Council. *Proposed performance procedures.* London: GMC, 1995.

General Medical Services Committee. *Annual report 1995: appendix III: interim report on individual reaccreditation.* London: GMSC, 1995.

Royal College of General Practitioners. *Portfolio-based learning in general practice: report of a working group on higher professional education.* London: RCGP, 1993.

Royal College of General Practitioners (Scottish Council). *Working party on reaccreditation in general practice: report to Scottish council.* Edinburgh: RCGP, 1993.

11 Audit and quality assurance

The recurrent theme of this book is the fact that postgraduate education for general practitioners has a wider dimension than just being "a good thing" for professionals to undertake. It has a direct connection with quality of practice and the expectations of members of the public of the doctors they consult.

There is a view that physicians who subscribe to a system that constantly questions their standards in terms of "knowledge, skills, and attitudes" would, of necessity, be practising to certain minimum standards. Such assumptions, however, are no longer thought to be sufficient in this age of accountability, and it is important that methods of testing parameters of quality are in place. These methods are listed in box 11.1

Box 11.1 Methods of quality assurance in British general practice

- Managerial methods
- Professional methods
- Methods involving *both* professional and managerial considerations

---

Quality assurance: management methods

Working for Patients, published by the government in 1989, was the document which heralded the major NHS reforms of

1990. It listed seven principal objectives, all of which were to do with improvement in the quality of service offered to patients either in hospitals or in the community.

One of the major criticisms of the reforms that flowed from *Working for Patients* was the intrusive style of management that was put in place, especially in general practice where "administrators" were transformed into "managers" almost overnight. Previously, general practitioners considered themselves to be the managers of their own practices, and many of them were already achieving the quality standards demanded of the new regimen. Thus much bureaucratic effort was required only to prove to the new style of primary care managers that quality in practice was indeed taking place, and the time spent in compiling reports and statistical returns was seen to be at the expense of clinical time spent with patients.

Box 11.2 Information demanded by the 1990 contract

- An annual report containing details of the partners, staff, and premises of a practice, together with details of patient referrals, the number of patients with certain chronic illnesses, and health promotion interventions and measurements
- Levels of target achievement for cervical cytology and childhood vaccinations
- Details of practice arrangements for a practice directory and for a practice leaflet
- Number of patients not seen for three years, number of patients eligible for an invitation for an "over 75" medical
- Details of a doctor's availability to see patients
- Information required to apply to be placed on minor surgery and child health surveillance lists

---

The 1990 contract, therefore, demanded new management effort of general practitioners and their practices and the categories of information required is listed in box 11.2 The list is not exhaustive, but criticisms of the 1990 contract are outside the scope of this book. One other aspect of the NHS reforms that *had* been requested by the profession was the introduction of systematic medical audit, and one of eight working papers published as part of the *Working for Patients* initiative was entirely on this subject.

Medical (or clinical) audit is seen by doctors primarily as a professional activity and is therefore covered properly in the next section. Management resources were made available, however, to foster its development and medical audit advisory committees (MAAGs) were established in all areas in England and Wales, with parallel structures in all the 15 health board areas of Scotland.

Medical audit in primary care has had to compete for resources from a pool which covers both hospital and general practice, and this has been further diluted by the extension of audit to all activity in the NHS including nursing and the professions allied to medicine. There is some feeling that primary care that looks after about 90% of all episodes of illness has perhaps not enjoyed an equitable share of those resources.

Quality assurance, patient's charters, and complaints

The new management ethos of the reformed NHS has also encouraged the achievement of quality by the promotion of patient's charters, which spell out minimum standards of quality to be expected, and by encouraging complaints if they are not met.

This type of approach, more usually found within commercial organisations than professional practices, has required fundamental change in doctors' attitudes but is an idea to which modern NHS managers appear firmly wedded.

The encouragement of complaints as a tool to enhance performance is also found difficult by doctors. Managers view complaints as expressions of opinion to be treasured and used as a vehicle for change; whereas most doctors still have an attitude that complaints are personal rejections and often herald a breakdown in a relationship.

Medical education, and more particularly education for medical management, is one way of helping doctors come to terms with this change in management style. Many courses have been constructed to help doctors manage their practices better and the GMSC has produced a whole raft of documents to contribute to this educational exercise. The royal college has also produced useful learning packages for management education.

The NHS executive (and the Scottish Council for Postgraduate Medical and Dental Education) has promoted many courses for doctors' management education, and while the funding arrangements discriminate against general practitioners there is a large amount of educational resource available to all doctors.

Being Heard, the report of the Wilson committee on complaints in the NHS was implemented in April 1996 and has major implications for general practice. Wilson has encouraged a common complaints procedure throughout the NHS, has separated complaints from disciplinary considerations, and has encouraged the resolution of the vast majority of complaints at a local or practice level without recourse to more formal procedures. Medical education will have a large part to play in the successful implementation of the Wilson report, and the government is has organised a training programme for key players at the time of writing.

Professional methods of quality assurance

There are several professional methods of quality assurance that are at least as important as those mediated by management interests. These are listed in box 11.3.

While NHS management has a vested interest in quality of service so too do doctors, for no other reason than their own professional standards and their desire to treat their patients effectively.

As described above, medical audit was one of the few professional desires of doctors actually delivered by the 1990 reforms, and, while some aspects of its implementation have

---

Box 11.3 Professional methods of quality assurance

- Medical or clinical audit
- Vocational training: assessment
- Accreditation of higher specialist training, trainer selection, and *What Sort of Doctor?*
- Standard setting, college membership and fellowship
- Standard setting, prescribing, complaints, and "three wise men"

Box 11.4 Medical audit as defined by *Working for Patients*

Medical audit is:

"the systematic, critical analysis of the quality of medical care, including the procedures used for diagnosis and treatment, the use of resources, and the resultant outcome and quality of life for the patient"

---

caused anxiety, the principle of a systematic examination of the quality of medical care has been generally welcomed. Medical audit is defined by *Working for Patients* as in box 11.4.

The connection of medical audit with education and training is twofold. Education in the basic principles and methods of medical audit is a general requirement of all new entrants to medical practice in all disciplines and is needed for those established practitioners whose basic training lacked such instruction. Secondly, the curriculum of postgraduate medical education can and should be informed by the results of audit.

The basic tasks inherent in applying medical audit as described by Marshall Marinker are listed in box 11.5.

The principal feature of medical audit is that it should not just be a research tool to find out what is happening within practice, it should be an engine for change and enhanced quality. A full description of the process of audit has filled many complete

---

Box 11.5 The basic tasks of medical audit (Marinker)

- Determining which aspects of current work are to be considered
- Describing and measuring present performance and trends
- Developing explicit standards
- Deciding what needs to be changed
- Negotiating change
- Mobilising resources for change
- Reviewing and renewing the process

Box 11.6 Summarises the conclusions of a report to the clinical outcomes group

Audit and quality assurance
This was a multidisciplinary group chaired by Sir Donald Irvine and gives a vision for audit and quality assurance in practice.

Audit and quality assurance in practice

- Achieving and maintaining good quality primary health care is most likely to happen where the practitioners who make up each practice unit are themselves committed to the philosophy, principles, and methods of quality assurance and quality improvement. NHS policy should therefore be directed unequivocally to this end
- Within each practice unit clinical audit should be regarded in future as an important tool of quality assurance and quality improvement rather than as an end in itself. Clinical audit embracing the cycle of standard setting, measurement against standards, and effecting and measuring change should be integrated fully within the general quality assuring arrangements of every practice unit
- Clinical audit should continue to be professionally led. It should "follow the patient" and so extend to any practitioner who is in some way involved with patients whose care is being assessed. Sometimes, therefore, clinical audit will be multidisciplinary, sometimes unidisciplinary, sometimes spanning the boundary between primary and secondary care or social services
- Practitioners and practices should be prepared to offer their work for external peer review
- Since the purpose of clinical audit is to improve patient care, the means will have to be found of engaging service users directly at all stages in the audit process wherever possible, so making the object of audit relevant to their needs and concerns
- In making clinical audit effective within each practice unit the greatest challenge will be in bringing the practitioners together regularly and successfully so that they can agree and commit themselves to their objectives and standards of care and any changes in practice policy and personal behaviour deemed necessary as a result of audit. Making multidisciplinary practice teams work effectively, and managing change constructively will be invariably more testing than mastering the technicalities of the audit process
- The central role of practice management in achieving effective teamwork and in the implementation of audit as part of wider quality assurance in primary health care must be fully acknowledged. Indeed we identify the improvement of management skills within individual practices as the highest priority area for immediate development
- Clinical audit should be based on good quality medical records arranged in an auditable format
- Clinical audit can be greatly facilitated by the full use of well designed computer systems. Further development of computer based systems is needed so that they may meet the requirements for primary health care and primary/secondary care audit. All practice units should have access to suitable training to ensure efficient data handling
- Clinical audit in primary health care should support the wider agenda for the development of primary health care services and also take into account the requirements set out by the NHS executive for clinical audit policy development throughout the NHS

textbooks, some of which are listed at the end of this chapter, and is beyond the scope of this book but a thumbnail sketch is given in box 11.6.

The contents of box 11.6 might be considered as a counsel of perfection and would not necessarily receive the support of all general practitioners. This is, however, a vision of how quality assurance might develop beyond the millennium.

Vocational training: assessment

Vocational training for general practice and both formative and summative assessment are covered in chapters 5 to 7. They are mentioned here for completeness and to reinforce the fact that the proper training, education, and regulation of standards of those aspiring to enter general practice are crucially important factors in the quality of practice delivered by its practitioners.

Accreditation of higher specialist training, trainer selection, and What Sort of Doctor?

Vocational training may be the "incubator", but equally important for quality are the educational standards, the teaching skills, and the practice environment offered by those appointed to carry out that education. Indeed, so important is the selection of trainers for general practice that it is the basis for the royal college's document *What Sort of Doctor*. This describes a method of assessment of the established general practitioner and the standards that would be expected at the end of a period of higher specialist training if this were ever to be introduced by the discipline and is largely predicated on the present structure of a trainer selection visit and the standards that are expected to be offered for inspection.

What Sort of Doctor defined several areas of performance and applied to each area several criteria for assessment. These are described in box 11.7.

Standard setting, college membership, and fellowship

The route to the MRCGP is also documented elsewhere (chapter 8). With the introduction of summative assessment of vocational training (chapter 7) and recent attempts by the royal college to align its examination with that process, there has been some debate as to the purpose and status of the MRCGP. Some believe that it should mark only the end point of vocational training, whereas many have always believed that it should be

Box 11.7

What Sort of Doctor*

Areas of performance	Criteria for Assessment
Professional values	Perception of role
	Responsibilities
	Personal care
	Development
	Professional growth
	Self awareness
	Personal behaviour
	Teaching and research
	Communication
	Patients' autonomy
	Professionalism
Accessibility	Consulting arrangements
	Home visits
	Patients' queries
	Contactability
	Out of hours cover
	Access to staff
	Facilitation
	Punctuality
Clinical competence	History taking
	Physical examination
	defining the problem
	Seeking further information
	Use of resources
	Explanation to the patient
	Management
	Prescribing
	Preventive medicine
	Continuing care
	Care of emergencies
Ability to communicate	Communication with the patient
	Communication with ancillary staff
	Communication with colleagues/team
	Referral letters
	Clinical records

* The *areas of performance* and *criteria for assessment* are given as headings only: further reading of the original document is recommended.

seen as a mark of quality and as an indicator of achievement of a standard of performance well above the minimum required for independent practice. We support the latter view, hence its inclusion in this chapter on quality in practice.

While the royal college is now attempting to abandon peer referencing of the examination and to base it more on criterion referencing, it is to be hoped that the standards it attests to are not to be devalued. Fellowship of the royal college, on the other hand, has always been concerned with standards deemed to be well above the mean, but there are now two routes to that status, only one of which has attached to it any degree of academic rigour.

The traditional route to fellowship has been that of recommendation by one's peer general practitioners, through the local faculty to a central committee at Princes Gate. The award of the fellowship is to recognise a significant contribution to the work of the college or the discipline, and while it is clear that it is supposed to be a mark of quality, it is awarded on fairly loose criteria and is essentially more a professional honour than an academic credential.

The second route to fellowship, now gradually gathering momentum, is fellowship by assessment. The assessment is largely based on the *What Sort of Doctor?* areas of performance and criteria of assessment described above (box 11.7). It is seen as a rigorous examination of a doctor's professional, clinical, and practice values and is a much prized award that truly recognises quality in practice.

Standard setting, prescribing, complaints, and "three wise men"

The royal college represents but one wing of general practice and might be regarded as the "academic" interest. The "service" wing of the profession, however, represented by the local medical committee or the general practitioner subcommittee of the area medical committee in Scotland, has an interest in quality also.

The quality and cost-effectiveness of prescribing has always been the preserve of the local medical committee and even though there are now medical prescribing advisers attached to health authorities, the supervisory role of the committee is still intact.

The service committee procedures that have existed since the inception of NHS general practice have also depended on peer review by local medical committee members, and even when they are superseded by the new arrangements under *Being Heard*, members will still maintain a role in maintaining quality by being involved in handling complaints and in the new disciplinary procedures to be introduced in April 1996.

There are occasions where matters of quality in practice cause sufficient concern that swift action is required by the profession to protect patients before the more formal, cumbersome action of GMC or NHS disciplinary machinery takes action. In these circumstances the "three wise men" procedure is often invoked.

The "three wise men" are usually senior office bearers of the local medical committee and will seek to counsel colleagues whose standards have slipped to such an extent that they should cease working until they can show that remedial action has again made them safe to practise.

Managerial/professional quality initiatives

One of the quality initiatives within the reformed NHS seems to have overtones of both professional and managerial credentials – the formulation and implementation of clinical guidelines and protocols.

Professional cooperation with compilation of guidelines stems from a recognition that not all clinical procedures are based on absolute scientific knowledge and principle and that the practise of evidence based medicine is an aim earnestly to be desired. The royal college has outlined six key points in its document, *The Development and Implementation of Clinical Guidelines*, these are listed in box 11.8.

In an NHS which is funded by public money, there will always be a clamour for the responsible use of those funds and for "value for money". The use of clinical guidelines, together with local protocols derived from them, is one method that management sees as legitimate to regulate more closely the use of resources by clinicians in the name of "clinical freedom".

So long as the guidelines are acceptable to the generality of doctors, they are not used solely as money saving devices, and they are regularly updated and do not stifle experimentation and innovation, it is likely that their use can become a point of agreement between doctors and management for the better care of patients. The educational input to clinical guidelines and protocols is derived from a systematic search of the available world literature and the intellectual exercise of sifting and evaluating such evidence.

Box 11.8 Key points in *The Development and Implementation of Clinical Guidelines*

- A central aim of guideline development and use should be to bring valid consensus to the practice of medicine, where this is justified by available scientific evidence and professional judgment
- Guidelines should therefore be generated by valid and reliable development processes
- Valid guidelines should be created by representative guideline development groups with a balance of skill appropriate to the task in hand
- Even valid guidelines will fail to benefit patients if distrusted or foisted on unwilling users or if presented inappropriately
- Guidelines should usefully carry an independent grading of validity, relevance, and practicability for the clinical setting of their intended use

---

Further reading

Marinker M, ed. *Medical audit and general practice*. London: BMJ Publishing, 1990.

Irvine D. *Managing for quality in general practice*. London: King's Fund Centre, 1990.

Irvine D, Irvine S, eds. *Making sense of audit*. Oxford: Radcliffe Medical Press, 1991.

Royal College of General Practitioners. *What sort of doctor? Assessing the quality of care in general practice*. London: RCGP, 1985.

Royal College of General Practitioners. *The development and implementation of clinical guidelines*. London: RCGP, 1995.

Department of Health. *Working for patients*. London: HMSO, 1989.

Department of Health. *Clinical outcomes group primary care clinical audit working group report to clinical outcomes group*. London: HMSO, 1995.

12 Academic general practice, undergraduate and postgraduate medical education, research

A narrow definition of academic general practice refers to general practice within the university system. In its wider sense, however, the definition refers to all those described under chapter 2.

Academic general practice in universities expanded mainly in the 70s and 80s and there is now a department in every university with a medical school in the United Kingdom. It has been a difficult development due to many factors, with the lack of a career structure being a particular problem. The Association of University Departments of General Practice (AUDGP) had a working party on career structure in 1993 when it concentrated on the concepts underpinning the development of an appropriate career structure. It recognised that there was a considerable number of practical, organisational, and financial issues which still needed to be debated and resolved, but in the report it dealt with principles and broad targets before dealing with the difficult process of implementation.

The report looked at a model for an academic career structure and how various career grades could be linked to particular levels of service and academic attainments. One recent innovation is the introduction of an academic registrar in general practice, which is a post which will require two years to be spent as a trainee general practitioner with half of that time spent in academic training. It was also thought important that all senior clinical academics should have principal status. The report thought that 10 years was a realistic time to reach the post of senior lecturer with 15 being more realistic for a chair. In academic practice there is a constant problem of how much time should be spent on each of the various components of research, clinical work, and teaching.

Clinical work – In the early parts of one's career 100% of time should be spent on clinical work and only after four to five years in the post of academic registrar should this be divided between half clinical and half academic. At senior lecturer level a one third/two third split between clinical and academic work seems appropriate with the academic work on promotion to a chair being 80% or over.

Research – We will return to this topic later in the chapter, but any doctor reaching the more senior academic posts would be expected to have either an MD or a PhD and to have published in peer reviewed journals

Teaching – Teaching experience would be expected at all stages of the academic ladder.

Box 12.1 Academic undergraduate general practice: main responsibilities

- Research
- Teaching
- Organisation
- Management

The association's working party recognised the need for a career structure which had built in flexibility. Not all general practitioners with academic aspirations make the decision early in their career to commit themselves to full time academic posts. Many of the current professors of general practice have a background of full time service general practice in their career years. Provided appropriate levels of academic and service attainment are reached the report did not express a preference between routes. It was thought that the creation of designated academic practices would be the lynchpin of future moves to broaden the academic base of general practice. A designated practice would have more teaching and research responsibilities but it would be envisaged that some practices might choose to be recognised for only one of the two functions. A fully designated academic practice, however, would:

- Contain one or more principals who are qualified to undertake research without supervision
- Be capable of providing training in research methods and in some cases supervising higher degrees
- Act as a clinical base for university employed academics in general practice
- Be a recognised training practice
- Conduct undergraduate and postgraduate teaching
- Provide higher clinical training for associate academic general practitioners.

Normally these practices would be independent but would have close links with their local university department.

Box 12.2 Designated academic practices

- Undertake research without supervision
- Provide training and research methods
- Act as clinical base
- Recognised training practice
- Conduct teaching
- Provide higher clinical training

In undergraduate departments the steps would be to complete vocational training and hopefully have principal status as a lecturer in general practice with definite principal status at the stages of senior lecturer and professor.

In postgraduate work doctors in the regional adviser structure have a much greater practice link; their academic work being almost wholly teaching and only a limited research base. This, however, is changing with regional advisers becoming full time appointments. The 1991 working party of the Conference of Regional Advisers in General Practice in England described the skill of the regional adviser as being in education, audit, and research, and this triad should provide the foundation on which postgraduate and continuing medical education develops. The regional adviser's major responsibility will continue to be as an academic in general practice with responsibility for vocational training, continuing medical education, medical audit and research.

Box 12.3 Responsibilities for regional advisers

- Vocational training
- Continuing medical education
- Medical audit
- Research

The separate development of university departments of general practice and those responsible for postgraduate training has created barriers to collaboration. This separation is impeding the academic development of the discipline and causes difficulties with recruitment and career progression. There is now a strong and widespread wish for those working in the undergraduate and postgraduate field to work together, and early steps are being taken to explore ways in which this could occur. Closer collaboration would establish a critical mass for research and educational development which would provide a stronger base for undergraduate, vocational, and higher professional training. Currently those in postgraduate education have little experience of research, and this makes movement between the undergraduate and the postgraduate areas difficult.

Structures throughout the United Kingdom differ greatly with some departments still having their own practice, but most are now practice linked for their clinical input.

Undergraduate and postgraduate medical education

In its document *Tomorrow's Doctors* the GMC has recognised that there would need to be a move to the health of populations, and public health and a shift from the hospital based services to those provided in general practice and the community. It also noted an aging population with changing patterns of disease and disability, and the application of new sciences and the increasing public understanding of disease and disability. In 1957, 1967, and 1980 the GMC had highlighted that the student's factual load should be reduced as far as possible to ensure that the memorising and reproduction of factual data should not be allowed to interfere with the 'primary need for fostering the critical study of principals and the development of independent thought. The student should also acquire and cultivate the ability to work independently. He or she must therefore have a certain amount of free time for private study and self education throughout the curriculum. These principles are the bases of many courses currently being set up throughout the United Kingdom.

Previously postgraduate education was unstructured and built on the apprenticeship model. With the development of vocational training which has been described elsewhere in the book, a structured approach is now very real with the current move towards self directed learning. This could change when the effects of the new curriculum progress into the postgraduate field, and this requires constant review as it develops.

Research

Research is a minority activity in general practice, and Howie, in his book *Research in General Practice*, emphasises that it is not a particularly difficult activity, although it does require the ability to think clearly and in an organised way. He also stated that it does not require extensive knowledge of experimental or statistical techniques nor the possession of an extensive vocabulary of specialised jargon. The volume of research work being carried out within the United Kingdom is increasing, and this is a credit to the Royal College of General Practitioners. With research it is important to read a basic text book like *Research in General Practice*, to ask questions which are important and require an answer, to have some degree of protected time to carry the work out, and to seek advice and to pilot at an early stage. Funding councils, noting the independent contractor status of the general practitioner, are now willing to fund protected time within a grant application. Time is important in carrying out research as is organisation and an eye for detail. When an idea is transformed into a research project it is important that a pilot study is carried out so that any methodological difficulties are revealed at an early stage.

A body of work in a specific area can be the basis for the proposal and completion of a higher degree. Advice regarding the mechanisms should be sought at an early stage from those within universities.

A higher degree forces a researcher to look at topics in much greater depth. For an MD, however, a question is the place to start and when one question has been answered another will almost certainly follow. When a series of questions are answered in a particular specialty then the basis is in place to plan an MD. A PhD would also be initiated in a similar way but is more likely to follow work already taking place within a department. This work could have some degree of funding with an element of supervision. MDs and PhDs in general practice are unusual, and around 100 of the 18 369 members of the royal college have a higher degree with 10 having both an MD and a PhD. The RCGP, however, has given the promotion of the doctoral thesis in general practice as one of their five current research priorities, and they regularly publish lists of doctors who have achieved a higher degree. The other four priorities are: to promote a culture of research in general practice; to establish research general practices; to establish as many research training fellowships as possible for general practitioners; and to foster an alliance among the academic organisations of general practice.

One way into research in general practice is to carry out an MSc under the supervision of a university department. The college now has a register of MSc courses provided by the academic departments of general practice throughout the United Kingdom. In addition, there are several general practice networks which can provide support for any aspiring researcher, and these are currently present in the northern region, the Midlands, Wessex and South Thames.

Further reading

General Medical Council. *Tomorrow's Doctors. Recommendations on undergraduate medical education.* London: GMC, 1993.

Working Party of the Association of University Departments of General Practice. *A career structure for academic general practice.* 1993.

Committee of Regional Advisers in General Practice in England. *The responsibilities of regional advisers.* 1991.

Howie JGR. *Research in general practice.* London: Chapman and Hall, 1989.

13 The European dimension: the Calman report and the European Union of General Practitioners

No description of postgraduate medical education for general practice would now be complete without mention of the influence of the United Kingdom's membership of the European Community (EC). No matter what decisions are taken within each member state with regard to the training of its doctors, they have to be made within the framework of the Treaty of Rome, the wider perspective of EC law, and the various directives adopted by the Council of Ministers.

This book is concerned primarily with *general* medical practice, however, at least two thirds of the training for the specialty currently takes place within hospital, and to understand the full implications of EC legislation on general practice it is necessary to examine its impact on doctors as a whole.

The directives relating to medical education in the United Kingdom are now consolidated in EC directive 93/16/EEC of 5 April 1993. The previous directives that it supersedes are listed in box 13.1.

These three consolidated directives have as their final intention: "To facilitate the free movement of doctors, and the mutual recognition of their diplomas, certificates and other evidence of formal qualifications" (93/16/EEC of 5 April 1993).

While the intention to produce European harmonisation is a

Box 13.1 European Community directives relating to medical education and training, now part of 93/16/EEC

- Directive 75/362/EEC: related to the mutual recognition of diplomas, certificates, and other evidence of formal qualifications in medicine; it also related to the exercise of the right of establishment of doctors from member states and the freedom to provide services
- Directive 75/363/EEC: related to the coordination of the legal framework for the activities of doctors and for the harmonisation between member states of basic and postgraduate training in the different specialties
- Directive 86/457/EEC: related to the setting up of vocational training in general practice as a first stage, and as a second stage made the practice of general practice conditional on the possession of a vocational training qualification

---

natural consequence of the United Kingdom's membership of a community of nations, the implications of its achievement have been no less in medicine than in any other aspect of life. United Kingdom citizens are often accused by others in Europe of having insular attitudes, and perhaps this is equally true of United Kingdom doctors. There is often a feeling that because the United Kingdom medical profession has developed its own traditions of medical education and training and its own, unique medical career structure that it is inherently superior to those traditions obtaining elsewhere in Europe. This may or may not be true, but there is now a legal imperative on the United Kingdom to move towards a structure that is congruent with that of our European neighbours.

The implementation of the European directives has brought about greatest change within education and training for hospital based specialties, and the threat of infraction procedures against the United Kingdom government was one of the main stimuli to the publication of the 1993 report *Hospital Doctors: Training for the Future.*This was the report of a working group on specialist medical training chaired by the chief medical officer of England (*The Calman Report*). The main recommendations of the Calman report are summarised in box 13.2:

Box 13.2 Recommendations of *Hospital Doctors: Training for the Future*: (the Calman report):

- The introduction of improved training programmes by the end of 1995
- The establishment of a single training grade by mid-1995 to replace career registrar and senior registrar grades
- The establishment of regular discussions between educational bodies and postgraduate deans
- The introduction of a new certificate of completion of specialist training (CCST)

Improved training programmes

One of the main anxieties of our European neighbours was the difference perceived between their "specialists" and holders of consultant posts in the United Kingdom. In the European sense, a "specialist" is a doctor who has satisfactorily completed training; such an achievement, however, does not guarantee the United Kingdom doctor automatic consultant status. In addition, there were great differences in the length of training in the United Kingdom for different specialties.

The Calman report suggested that all medical royal colleges should develop more organised training programmes, while maintaining standards, seize the opportunity for a significant reduction in the duration of training, and for such training to be completed within a period of seven years.

To this end a subgroup was set up to examine the various specialist training programmes and to advise the chief medical officer on the changes required to bring the United Kingdom into line with EC law, especially with regard to the structure, duration, standards, and quality of that training.

A single training grade

The Calman subgroup recognised that one of the main factors contributing to the inordinate length of specialist training was "the lack of opportunities for doctors to advance both within the training grades and on completion of training." The ability to shorten training was constrained by the training grade structure and hence its recommendation to amalgamate the career registrar and senior registrar grades into what has become known as the specialist registrar grade. Thus an individual's progress would be entirely dependent on educational achievement and not on the availability of suitable promoted posts.

Regular discussions between postgraduate deans and educational bodies

Under new arrangements, postgraduate deans have become the "managers" of medical education. The regular discussions suggested by Calman, through existing committee mechanisms, served as a catalyst for discussion of the crucial issues of training standards and the relation between service and training requirements among the "stakeholders" involved – medical royal colleges, the NHS management executive, established specialists, and doctors in training.

The certificate of completion of specialist training (CCST)

Calman recommended that when a doctor has satisfactorily completed the training prescribed by a medical royal college, he or she should be awarded the certificate of completion of specialist training by the competent authority for the United Kingdom – the GMC on the advice of the relevant royal college.

The award of this certificate would give a doctor two rights: the right to free movement within the EC with the status of "specialist" and the right to apply for a consultant post within the NHS. The intention of this recommendation was to recognise that a doctor can satisfactorily complete specialist training, thus bringing him or her into line with a European counterpart. This would not necessarily accord the doctor the status of an NHS consultant, however, which would remain an appointment with special privileges made only after a competitive selection process.

Calman and "non-hospital" careers

The thumbnail sketch given above of new educational and training arrangements for that 50% of doctors who enter hospital practice does not cover the special arrangements that would have to apply to three remaining groups of United Kingdom doctors: general practitioners, overseas graduates, and academics. The original Calman report also recognised this deficiency and three supplementary working groups were established. The only one of direct relevance to this book is the *Supplementary Report on the*

Box 13.3 Recommendations of the working group on implications of the Calman report for general medical practice

The length of vocational training and the relative duration of the hospital and general practice components of training

- Two phases of training: a period of vocational training and a voluntary period of higher/further training/education
- Definition of required competencies for both phases
- Attainment of core competencies in vocational training to be the minimum requirement for trainees entering general practice
- Flexibility in the balance of training between hospital and general practice
- A specific provision for the enhancement of training within primary care within any transfer of resources from secondary to primary care

Assuring the educational quality of senior house officer posts

- Greater understanding of the relative values of the hospital and general practice components of vocational training and better cooperation between them
- Improvements to the training programmes for all senior house officers
- Review of the selection procedure for senior house officer posts for vocational training
- GMC to take account of general practice in its recommendations on general professional training
- Variation of the duration of hospital posts to encourage flexible training

Assessment methods for vocational trainees

- Demonstration of competence in specified areas to an agreed national standard before entry to general practice
- Relevant certification for locums, deputies, and assistants before undertaking NHS general practice in line with EC directive 93/16/EEC

Opportunities for general practitioner experience for hospital trainees

Exploitation of the contribution of academic general practice

Development of an integrated plan for the career development of general practitioner educators

Funding arrangements for vocational training

- Transfer of resources to purchase vocational training to postgraduate deans' budgets
- Regional advisers, working with postgraduate deans, empowered to purchase suitable training opportunities

Implications for General Medical Practice, finally published in May 1995.

The main recommendations of the general practice supplementary report are summarised in box 13.3.

The length of vocational training

As far back as 1966 the royal college submitted evidence to the royal commission on medical education (the Todd report) that there should be a five year training period for general practice, and this recommendation was accepted in a modified form when Todd reported in 1968. When the vocational training regulations were laid, however, a compromise period of three years of training after full registration was prescribed.

The job description of the British general practitioner has expanded dramatically in the intervening 30 years, and there are now strong opinions that the training period should be lengthened. With the advent of summative assessment (see below) these arguments might not now be so valid because training beyond a defined level of competence can not, of itself, be justified. There is general agreement among general practitioner educationalists, however, that the balance of training between hospital and practice is wrong and that there needs to be a longer time spent in that working environment for which the doctor is training.

Assessment of training implies the compilation of a curriculum for the discipline so that assessors know what to assess – hence the recommendation that a list of "core competencies" is defined, that they should be attained, and that there should be flexibility between hospital and practice in their attainment.

Resources are required for any educational process, and Calman recommended that some of those should be derived from a transfer from the secondary sector of health care.

Assuring the quality of senior house officer posts

The most consistent criticism of vocational training over the years has been the inconsistent quality of training within the hospital component, and Calman has made several specific recommendations to deal with this long standing problem.

Assessment methods for vocational trainees

The Calman report was written at a time when formative (educational) assessment of vocational training was just beginning to be universally introduced and when summative (regulatory) assessment was being slowly developed in only a few regions.

This work was recognised and commended by the report, which took the view that there should be a minimum standard shown by all doctors working within the discipline. Assessment is described in depth in chapter 7.

Opportunities for general experience for hospital trainees

In 1948 the profession was effectively divided between those working exclusively in the community as general practitioners and those spending their entire careers within hospitals. Ever since that rather artificial division there has been a feeling among many that it led to a certain loss of perspective among hospital practitioners about how illness relates to individual patients and their families. Many hospital doctors who have spent even a short time within general practice have thought that it has helped them in their professional development, and Calman has suggested that such an opportunity should be offered to all medical graduates, whatever their eventual career destination.

Exploitation of the contribution of academic general practice and development of an integrated plan for the career development of general practitioner educators

Calman has recognised that any medical discipline needs its own corpus of knowledge and research to sustain its intellectual development. The report recommends more explicit use of the educational and research resources resident in academic general practice.

Funding arrangements for vocational training

The Calman report has acknowledged the concept of "the market" and "purchasers and providers" inherent to the 1990 NHS reforms and has made recommendations that accord with that philosophy. Some elements of the profession are uncomfortable with these concepts, believing that there is a danger in according too much power to academic structures; these new arrangements, however, seem likely to be adopted by the NHS management. (The financial and professional accountability arrangements exclusive to the Scottish Council for Postgraduate Medical and Dental Education are described in chapter 2.)

European Union of General Practitioners (UEMO)

With the development of the European Community various medical organisations have developed to foster international co-operation among European doctors and to represent a consensus to the Council of Ministers and the European Commission when European health policy is determined. The European Union of General PractitionersP (UEMO), founded in 1967, deals with general practitioners' European interests and since 1972 general practitioners in the United Kingdom have been represented at UEMO by the BMA.

Since its foundation UEMO has made several important policy statements, including those in specific areas such as criteria for GP trainers, therapeutic prescriptions, computerised medical records, continuing medical education, quality assurance in general practice, and cancer training for general practitioners. The most important policy statement in the context of postgraduate medical education, however, was UEMO's *Consensus document on specific training for general practice*, which was unanimously adopted at its conference in Copenhagen in October 1994. (The EC now refers to vocational training for general practice as "specific training".)

Box 13.1 describes the EC directives relating to medical education and training, and these are now consolidated in directive 93/16/EEC. This directive obliged member states to harmonise various aspects of training, to introduce mutual

---

Box 13.4 UEMO consensus document on specific training for general practice

The main subjects covered by the document include:
- The training required
- The medical job description of the general practitioner (preventing, diagnosing, curing, and caring)
- The wider dimension of general practice (psychological and social aspects of illness and the preservation of health)
- The unique attributes of the trained general practitioner and his/her contribution to the wider health care system
- The ideal system for specific (or vocational) training in terms of location, length, content, and quality

---

Box 13.5 List of recommendations concerning specific (vocational) general practice training (UEMO, 1994)

- General practitioners should be in charge of all aspects and elements of training, whether undertaken in or outside general practice
- All doctors should be exposed to general practice training both as undergraduates and as part of postgraduate training before entering a specialty
- Specific (vocational) training must be general practitioner oriented throughout the entire training period
- Specific (vocational) training must be of a minimum duration of *three years*
- Training should produce a general practitioner with a level of competence sufficient for independent practice
- At least 50% of training must be spent in the general practice environment
- EC directives governing general practice should in future apply to all general practitioners, not just those practising within a social security system
- Quality of training must be delivered through explicit contracts specifying educational content and mechanisms for evaluation
- The time spent in part time training should be at a minimum of 50% of full time training (not the current minimum of 60%)
- There must be the promotion of research methodology and quality assurance in general practice during training
- Methods of evaluation must be intrinsic to training programmes
- There must be the provision of sufficient and substantial resources for specific (vocational) training
- A common core content of training should be defined throughout Europe preparing general practitioners for independent practice in all European countries
- General practitioners migrating to another member state may need to have additional training available to familiarise them with the conditions of practice in the host country
- Manpower planning for general practice is needed in each member state to avoid overproduction of general practitioners and possible migratory imbalance

recognition of that training, and to set minimum standards for the right to practise as a general practitioner. The European Commission is committed to review the implementation of the directive by 1 January 1996, and UEMO has evolved this consensus statement in the context of this review, the result of which is still awaited.

The main conclusions of the Copenhagen conference included in the consensus document are summarised in box 13.4.

Given that this is a consensus document the list of recommendations is remarkably specific, and it should have a major impact on the future direction for general practice in the United Kingdom. The recommendations are listed, without elaboration, in box 13.5. There is a little doubt among educators in this country that implementation of these European policies would solve many of the current problems in education and training for general practice in the United Kingdom.

Further reading

European Union of General Practitioners (UEMO). *Proceedings: UEMO consensus conference on specific training for general practice, including cancer training for general practitioners.* Copenhagen: Danish Medical Association for UEMO, 1995.

Department of Health. *Hospital doctors: training for the future: the report of the working group on specialist medical training.* Manchester: Health Publications Unit, 1993.

Department of Health. *Hospital doctors: training for the future: a supplementary report by the working group commissioned to consider the implications for general medical practice arising from the principal report.* Manchester: Health Publications Unit, 1995.

European Union of General Practitioners (UEMO). *European Union of general practitioners reference book 1995/96* London: Kensington Publications/UEMO, 1995.

14 Technical innovations in postgraduate medical education

Traditional medical education has been based on three teaching and learning styles that are still used today but on a steadily diminishing basis; these are:

- Learning from textbooks
- The traditional, didactic lecture
- Bedside teaching/learning.

Each of these styles of education have their disadvantages, but common to the first two is the lack of interaction between teacher and learner. The third is the very basis of the apprenticeship model which many hold dear and thankfully is still possible within the general practice training year for vocational training. Bedside teaching within hospitals or when used for continuing medical education, however, is not very successful unless performed with very small numbers of students. Useful bedside teaching is therefore extravagant in its use of teaching resources and, with increasing pressure on clinicians' time, is becoming more and more difficult to organise.

In more recent times the concept of small group teaching has gained ground which requires new skills of teachers concerned with the psychology of group dynamics and with personal skills of facilitation. Most traditional medical educators possessed vast amounts of expert knowledge, and such knowledge is still demanded of modern teachers. There is, however, a need for

139

special educational attributes for a small group leader to cope with the uncertainty of a wide ranging and unfocussed discussion and with the need to encourage contributions from the more introverted members of a group.

Given the disadvantages of traditional methods of education, technology has made possible an interactive form of education without the need for doctors always to meet in groups or, if they do, has provided resources greater than that of one, individual, talented educator. The new educational resources are summarised in box 14.1.

Box 14.1 New educational resources and teaching

- Distance learning packages
- Education based on information technology
- Computer assisted learning

Distance learning packages

In some respects distance learning has always been present in the form of the printed word, and medical textbooks were introduced almost at the same time as the invention of the printed word by Caxton in the sixteenth century. Even despite the explosion of electronic publishing in the past few years, the printed word in the form of standard textbooks and medical journals is still the fundamental basis of medical knowledge.

In more recent times, many medical journals have introduced questionnaires within their printed text so that the reader can test the knowledge acquired, and this is the first example of an interaction in its crudest form between the author and the reader.

Over the past decade newer forms of publishing have emerged which are based much more explicitly on this interaction, and at the end of every section or module the reader is tested in a formative way so that the degree of assimilation of new information is fed back to the student.

The centre for medical education at the University of Dundee has been in the forefront of these developments and has particularly concerned itself with the education of general practitioners, many of whom practice at a considerable distance from recognised centres of learning.

During the 1980s the Royal College of General Practitioners established its *Continuing Learning in Practice Project*. Part of that project was the CASE programme (clinical assessment for systematic education), which was set up in association with Dundee University with financial help from the pharmaceutical industry. The programme reached some 10 000 of the general practitioners in the United Kingdom (about one third of the total) and requests for distribution were received from 18 countries throughout the world. The programme consisted of a series of clinical vignettes with a choice of several therapeutic or management actions attached to each. The choices of the student were able to be compared instantly with the decisions of 50 established general practitioners and with that of a recognised specialist. At the end of the booklet a list of "key points" for the subject under review was provided.

A development of this concept was represented by a more recent programme, again developed by the University of Dundee sponsored by the (then) Scottish Council for Postgraduate Medical Education (SCPME) - the 1988 programme active continuing education (ACE). In this a series of clinical or management problems was developed by a team of working general practitioners and presented in a loose leaf binder. The programme was given a realistic "feel" to it by reproducing facsimiles of clinical notes, doctors' letters, clinical photographs, radiographs, etc, and even included audiotapes of doctors' conversations discussing the problems under review.

The programme had a double advantage as a distance learning package – it could be used by an individual, but it was an even better resource for a small number of doctors working as a group. Because of the realistic nature of the material and its comprehensive inclusion of questions and of pauses with set discussion points the need for an expert facilitator was avoided.

Distance learning has been accepted as a device for achievement of credits for the postgraduate educational allowance (see chapter 10). This recognition was given in acceptance of the fact that those doctors who are most remote from postgraduate centres would have greater difficulty and expense in achievement of allowances. Distance learning, however, perhaps ironically, is shunned by remote doctors probably because what they crave most in their professional isolation is social and intellectual intercourse with other doctors. Despite this fact, distance learning remains a useful resource for any busy doctor and its interactive nature ensures that not only is the printed word read but that it impinges on the consciousness!

Information technology based education

The expression "IT" means computers to most doctors. Computer assisted learning is mentioned specifically in the next section but IT can mean more than merely using a learning package on a computer.

Medical education, of course, is based on the accumulated knowledge and wisdom of many other doctors practising worldwide. One of the main uses of IT is its ability to find, retrieve, and handle large amounts of information.

Every doctor has experience of spending many hours in a medical library searching for relevant references in *Index Medicus* to inquire into an area of medical knowledge. In the 1990s access to a personal computer is almost universal, and, together with a modem, the computer now allows the doctor access to a medical database anywhere in the world where there is a telephone line and another computer.

The BMA library *Medline* service is the best known in this country and allows BMA members free access to a computerised version of *Index Medicus* and most general practitioners now have the ability to access up to date information from their home or surgery. Other services are available commercially and offer similar access to medical databases.

The Internet is now also generally available and permits access to a vast amount of information held on different computers worldwide. Originally developed to link the defence interests of the United States with its various universities and institutions of higher learning, the Internet is the most obvious example of the "information explosion" now facing society in the late twentieth century. This information is not available exclusively to doctors, however, but also to their increasingly well informed patients, and this opportunity for doctors to keep their medical knowledge up to date is fast becoming a professional necessity.

Alongside computers the other "arm" of IT is telecommunications. Fibreoptic cables and ISDN telephone lines are now capable of transmitting vast amounts of digitised information, and images and sound are now able to be carried, almost without distortion, around the world.

This has now made possible the transmission of radiographs, television and photographic images, and high quality sound. The United States Army is already developing surgery for the battlefield by using high quality, three dimensional images and sophisticated computer robotics software, making it possible for a surgeon to operate on a patient a long way away from a field hospital. In addition, training for surgery is now possible with computer simulation rather than using real patients for the better development of surgical technique. This same technology also has potential use for remote consultations, and there are already examples of dermatological consultations being conducted by transporting television images down telephone lines.

The implications of these developments for medical education are obvious to those who practise many miles from centres of excellence and may herald a new method of serving the educational needs of those in rural areas where educational activities are brought to them by IT rather than doctors having to travel. Despite the advantages, the same need for people to meet and discuss matters on a one to one basis will still exist, and such innovation is likely to meet the same resistance as more mundane forms of distance learning as described above.

Computer assisted learning

The best known form of this type of learning, which has been used for some years, is the *phased evaluation programme* (PEP). This was developed by the south east faculty of the royal college and has been issued freely to general practitioners all over the United Kingdom, with a more general use in the medical branch of the armed forces, who have used it extensively as a method of formative assessment.

The programme is really an electronic form of the multiple choice question examination but uses high quality images, sound, colour, and the versatility of computer software to secure its educational function. Rather like the CASE and ACE programmes mentioned above the evaluation programme presents the student with a clinical scenario and demands a reaction to a diagnostic, therapeutic, or management problem. Its highly visual impact brings a great sense of reality to bear and is as near as the student can get to a problem short of "virtual reality" software or a real, live patient. Once a choice is made from the menu offered the student can be congratulated on a correct choice or directed to a more appropriate one with supplementary information to reinforce existing knowledge or to correct erroneous opinion.

A special feature of most programmes is a preliminary exploration of students' confidence in various areas of knowledge with a feedback of actual performance for later comparison. Improving trends can be charted over the time of an educational course, and a comparison with one's peers who have also subscribed to the programme is possible. This is truly formative assessment.

Other recent technical innovations have included special television programmes broadcast in a scrambled form in the middle of the night which, with the aid of a video recorder and a special decoder, can be replayed at a doctor's leisure. Such programmes have few advantages over the distribution of videotapes. Development of cable television promises the possibility of interactive television programmes which could work similarly to the programme described above.

The future

The pace of change of technology is accelerating year on year. Black and white television is still in the recall of at least half of today's practising doctors, and the power of a modern desktop computer required a large room to house it a mere 20 years ago.

The development of new generations of software, new telecommunication technology, and the fast advancing science of robotics make the description of the future shape and scope of medicine almost impossible to predict. All that is certain is that the enormous changes seen in practice since the foundation of the NHS in 1948 will be as nothing to the change that today's medical graduates will see in their professional lifetime. Medical education will have to grasp all this technological advance to equip modern doctors with the knowledge and training they will require to be able to continue to practise effectively.

15 The future: a look into the 21st century

The years 1948, 1966, and 1990 all produced landmark changes to general practice. On each occasion the discipline of general practice moved further from traditions that have been in place since the mid-Victorian era. Change is therefore accelerating and is reflecting an equal change in the pattern of British society and of the lifestyles of the patients who general practitioners serve. To predict the future is always dangerous because it is necessarily hypothetical. There are underlying trends already established, however, that can inform the process, and the only certainty that exists is that the status quo will not remain.

Engines of change

The various factors that have produced and will continue to produce change in society, and consequently on general medical practice, are summarised in box 15.1.

Consumerism in society

In the last quarter of the twentieth century the role of the professional has faced a considerable onslaught from consumerism – a concept born in the United States, advocated by articulate exponents such as Ralph Nader, and grasped and exploited by the conservative governments of Margaret Thatcher and John Major.

The philosophy of consumerism has changed the NHS almost out of recognition and promoted the "patient" from the position of a supplicant for state health benefits to that of "valued customer". Consequently, doctors in the reformed NHS are no longer powerful and omnipotent agents of a government funded

145

Box 15.1 Engines of change

- Consumerism in society
- Increasing levels of general education
- Public access to information and information technology
- Demographic change
- Necessity to ration health care and doctors as "gatekeepers"
- The commissioning process
- Changes in professional roles and skill mix
- Transfer of care from the secondary sector
- Guidelines, protocols, and "evidence based" medicine
- Availability of new diagnostic and therapeutic technology

---

service answerable only to their own professional codes. They are now seen by many as mere providers of a service purchased on the customer's behalf by a multiplicity of the small, local businesses, which health authorities have now become in the eyes of the NHS executive.

This view, of course, is extreme and uncomfortable to many older doctors and may be reversed to some extent as the flavour of future governments change. What is most unlikely, however, is a return to the previously unchallenged position of doctors as absolute arbiters of patient care in the NHS.

Increasing levels of general education

Even with a diminution in the power of consumerism doctors will never again be placed on the kind of pedestal they occupied previously because the members of the public whom they treat are now much better educated. They have a better level of basic education at school, a far higher proportion are entering tertiary education, and even those who do not are constantly exposed to the mass media which frequently place medical matters high on their priority list for programming.

Even the more traditional printed media are now issuing an ever increasing number of publications dedicated to health, fitness, and lifestyle issues, and the public's demand for such information seems insatiable.

Public access to information and information technology

While the mass media are planning a huge expansion in their

ability to reach and inform the public by the development of multiple channel satellite and cable broadcasting, which promises the ability to summon medical information almost at will, a newer technology is growing fast. Britain has the highest per capita ownership of personal computers in the Western world, and modem connection to a ubiquitous telephone network will bring about ever greater access to information.

The Internet was developed in the United States as a method of connecting government defence agencies, centres of higher learning, and central databases. This network has now grown to the extent that almost any information is available to the domestic computer owner. The time is not far away when a patient will attend a doctor with as much up to date information about a medical condition drawn down from the Internet as is available to the professional he or she is consulting. Such a situation is intimidating for the doctor and, for the patient, possibly dangerous because of the considerable potential for misinterpretation of that information. Medical education will have to be adapted to cope with this eventuality.

Demographic change

Britain and the Western world generally is now supporting an aging population, which will continue to age well into the next century. An aging population means that the pattern of disease will change and, because of the nature of geriatric medicine, will mean that multiple pathologies will often be exhibited in the same patient. Because of current policies to move the care of elderly patients into "the community" and away from institutions, the general practitioner of the future will have to be far more expert in the diagnosis and treatment of the ailments of old age. This, again, will have implications for medical education.

Necessity to ration health care and doctors as "gatekeepers"

· The needs of an aging population, together with increasingly expensive treatments becoming available, will mean that doctors will have to become "gatekeepers" in more than name. Fundholding, brought in by the 1990 reforms, is a first step along this road as it empowers general practitioners to make purchasing decisions for a defined population of patients, but these decisions have to be made within the constraints of a fixed and finite budget.

It would only be proper for "rationing" decisions to be made in the context of a full public debate, such as was attempted in Oregon in the 1980s, but at the end of the day one individual clinician will have to make a decision. General practitioners will need training in health economics, and medical education will have an even more important role in this sphere in the future.

The commissioning process

The *rationing* of care is the extreme example; even to manage a purchasing strategy property and to commission the routine care of a population, however, will needs skills of a general practitioner more usually found in the discipline of public health medicine.

The current fundholding scheme may flourish and become the model for the future, but many health economists feel that the size of populations on which it is presently predicated are too low, and their size is certainly smaller than that of the health maintenance organisations that have flourished in the United States.

Perhaps a more likely scenario is the development of a hybrid model involving both fundholding and locality commissioning. What is now clear is that the general practitioner is moving away from being solely a diagnostician and therapist and is now increasingly adopting the role of a "manager of care". This commissioning activity will also require dedicated training and education to foster the skills that will be needed.

Changes in professional roles and skill mix

There is a perception that general practitioners are "over-skilled" for many of the tasks they currently undertake. The treatment of routine upper respiratory tract infections, cuts, bruises, aches, pains – and even more complicated conditions such as the care of stable asthmatics or diabetics – is well within the competence of trained nurses. Indeed, many practice nurses are already carrying out such tasks, albeit under close supervision.

It is indeed possible that in the future the general practitioner will become "the general physician" of yesteryear, previously based in hospitals, and act more in a consultant capacity to other members of the primary health care team.

Transfer of care from the secondary sector

As mentioned above, this transfer is already taking place. The frail elderly patient, the long term mentally ill, and those with special learning needs have already been decanted to the care of the general practitioner. In addition, patients having acute surgery or those recovering from serious incidents such as myocardial infarction are spending less and less time within hospitals, and the general practitioner is now required to exhibit different and enhanced skills. This process shows no sign of slowing and is likely to increase even further especially if the general practitioner becomes "the general physician in the community".

Guidelines, protocols, and "evidence based" medicine

Variation of standard of care and variation in health costs have always been a concern of government, which eventually meets the cost of the NHS through taxation. A recent concentration on the development of national guidelines based on the best available medical evidence for the efficacy of treatment, together with local implementation in the form of protocols, is seen as the way forward.

There are considerable professional worries over such an approach, largely concerned with loss of clinical freedom, rigidity of practice, and loss of innovation and possible medicolegal implications, but it would seem that evidence based medicine is here to stay. General practitioners will need special education to help to understand, develop, implement, and change guidelines and protocols in the future.

Availability of new diagnostic and therapeutic technology

A principal reason for admission in the past has always been that hospitals are where sophisticated technical facilities are sited. With increasing development of miniaturisation, electronic innovation, digitisation of information, and telemetry, however, there will be much less reason in the future for the patient to attend a hospital centre.

Given that much more equipment will be available to the general practitioner in years to come, education and training will have to be tailored to utilise the opportunities that will arise.

Medical education for the new millennium

The paragraphs above concerning the "engines of change" give some indication of the new demands that will be made of a future system of medical education. Information technology and access to the Internet is seen as a possible resource for patients, but it must be even more important for general practitioners, especially those remote from centres of learning. Computers also have a unique ability to develop interactive learning, amply demonstrated by the phased evaluation programme (PEP) already in existence. Extension of the broadcast media is also already being used and encrypted medical programmes are presently being broadcast through the night to doctors' video recorders. There is potential for enhanced use of this medium, together with dedicated medical cable television services.

Evidence based medicine will be as important to general practice as to any other specialty, and given that hospitals are seeing disease over a steadily diminishing time scale, observations of those diseases and their treatments within community settings will be crucial.

The *methods* of disseminaton of education can be discussed speculatively, however the single most important factor in the medical education of the future will be its *curriculum*. New skills to deal with an aging, better informed, articulate practice population will become essential. Enhanced training in the diagnosis and management of disease, without having to rely so much on hospital resources, will be another necessary component. Training in health needs assessment and the deployment of resources, together with a background in epidemiology will need to develop. Computer literacy, skills in team building and management, practice management and an ability to delegate to others are all part of the education of the future.

Finally, and most importantly, all these skills will have to be taught in the context of a continuing commitment to the professionalism that we presently hold so dear and which were restated in the 1994 BMA conference on core values. If general practitioners become efficient health economists, planners, diagnosticians, therapists, and "Internet surfers" – but forget their duty to be the patient's personal physician, advocate, and friend – the future looks bleak indeed. While at the end of the twentieth century one must recognise the uncertainties that beset society as a whole, and doctors in particular, however, equally one must take comfort from the enthusiasm, industry, and dedication shown by those who follow. The conference on core values showed that doctors from across the spectrum of age and specialty still subscribe to the intrinsic professional ethos that has driven physicians from ancient times. "Knowledge, skills, and attitudes" has become almost a cliché in medical writing but, together with self regulation, they still form the kernel of our professionalism and with this book's examination of general practitioner postgraduate education in terms of another near cliché, "structure, process, and outcome" one can be confident of the future health of the discipline.

Index